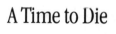

A Time to Die

CHARLES F. MCKHANN, M.D.

A Time to Die

The Place for Physician Assistance

YALE UNIVERSITY PRESS / NEW HAVEN & LONDON

Designed by Nancy Ovedovitz and set in Simoncini Garamond type by The Composing Room of Michigan, Inc. Printed in the United States of America.

Library of Congress Cataloging-in-Publication Data

McKhann, Charles F.

A time to die : the place for physician assistance / Charles F. McKhann.

    p.   cm.

Includes bibliographical references and index.

ISBN 0-300-07631-2 (alk. paper)

1. Assisted suicide. I. Title

R726.R355 1999

179.7—dc21   98-22193

A catalogue record for this book is available from the British Library.

The paper in this book meets the guidelines for permanence and durability of the Committee on Production Guidelines for Book Longevity of the Council on Library Resources.

10 9 8 7 6 5 4 3 2 1

To Rhona,
who is everything

Contents

Acknowledgments

It is unfortunate that I cannot cite by name the people who contributed the most to make this book possible, the many patients and their families who shared precious twilight hours with me. Their willingness to let me explore the most sensitive subjects with them and the candor with which they expressed their hopes and their fears were an education for me and provided much of the material upon which this book is based. Immediately behind the patients themselves are the physicians who took care of them, most of whom are my colleagues on the faculty at Yale Medical School. Again, many hours of thoughtful discussion will be easily recognized in the following pages. Although most of the physicians remain anonymous in the text, it is a pleasure to acknowledge them by name here: from the Department of Medicine, Doctors Wen-Jen Poo, Jill Lacy, David Fischer, Michael Reiss, John Marsh, Ken Marek, Dennis Cooper, Arthur Levy, John Murren, Louis Koldjcan, Ann Berger, Joel Wirth,

Richard Matthay, Alan Kliger, and Eric Brown; from the Department of Surgery, Doctors Marc Lorber, John Baldwin, Stephen Cohn, Gerard Burns, and Daniel Lowe; from the Department of Psychiatry, Doctors James Ciarcia and Claudia Bemis; from the Department of Gynecology, Dr. Peter Schwartz; from the Department of Hematology, Dr. Thomas Duffy; and from the Department of Radiation Therapy, Dr. Richard Peschel.

Four nurses also shared their experiences with me: Anna Peterson, R.N.; Karen Coombs, R.N.; Barbara Fusell, R.N.; and Mary Zorzanello, R.N. I also appreciate the input of several chaplains affiliated with Yale–New Haven Hospital: Rev. Omar Alamonte, Rev. James Schumake, Rev. Margaret Edgerly, Rev. Alan Mermann (who is also chaplain to Yale Medical School), Rabbi Stephen Steinberg, and Father Raymond Barry, as well as Rabbi Michael Whitman of Young Israel Temple, New Haven.

Yale–New Haven Hospital administrators Edwin Cadman, M.D., John McNeff, and attorney Virginia Roddy talked to me about the financial and legal aspects of assisted dying from the hospital's point of view. The history and goals of the Hemlock Society were provided by Midge Levy, Faye Girsh, and John Pridonoff. Similar information about Compassion in Dying came from Rev. Ralph Mero, Susan Dunshee, Thomas Preston, M.D., and attorney Kathryn Tucker.

At greater distance, a number of people in Holland were more than helpful in explaining to me the system that they have evolved: Adrian J. F. M. Kerkhof, Robert J. Dillmann, Paul J. van der Maas, Loes Pijnenborg, Gerrit van der Wal, Wilfred S. van Oijen, M. M. Calff, Gerrit K. Kimsma, and two unforgettable families who spent hours recounting their experiences with me. British views on assisted dying were explained to me by John Oliver, general secretary of the Voluntary Euthanasia Society, and by Professor Andrew Grubb of the Center for Medical Law and Ethics, King's College, London. My understanding of the legal aspects of assisted dying was augmented by Michael Reisman and Robert Burt of Yale Law School,

Gayle Westerman of Pace University Law School, David Orentlich er of Indiana University Law School, Ronald Dworkin of New York University and Oxford University Law Schools, and Kathryn Tucker, counsel for Compassion in Dying in Seattle. Ann Alpers and Mark Heilig discussed the attitudes of physicians and patients toward assisted dying in San Francisco.

Very special thanks go to Howard Spiro, M.D., at Yale, for reviewing part of the manuscript, to Margaret Battin of the Department of Philosophy at the University of Utah for discussing the project on many occasions and providing introductions to her colleagues in Holland, and to William Winslade, professor of philosophy in medicine at the University of Texas, Galveston, for reviewing the entire manuscript and providing many helpful suggestions. I am also grateful to Alex Hoffman, former publisher of Doubleday, for his suggestions and unflagging interest. My in-house editor, who also introduced me to the many "colours" of the English language, is my wife, Rhona. The manuscript was prepared by the nimble mind and hands of Maureen Scranton and was guided through the halls of Yale University Press by Jean Thomson Black.

Finally, the entire project was made possible by the generous support of the Rudkin Family Foundation and the personal interest of two members of the family, William and Henry Rudkin.

A Time to Die

Dying is personal. And it is profound. For many, the thought of an ignoble end, steeped in decay, is abhorrent. A quiet, proud death, bodily integrity intact, is a matter of extreme consequence. *Justice William Brennan*

Introduction

This book is about physician-assisted dying, which I think is both desirable and inevitable. Already much of the public is in favor of it, as are many physicians. Recent court decisions have so highlighted the diversity of thought on this issue that many people question whether there is—or needs to be—an absolute right or wrong. As the states have been encouraged by the courts to enact their own laws, so, too, have individuals been essentially freed to reach their own conclusions, to discuss them with their physicians, and even to act upon them.

My interest in physician-assisted dying and the earliest impetus to write this book grew out of my father's death in one of the best hospitals in the country. A physician himself, he died in 1988, at the age of eighty-nine, with widespread intra-abdominal cancer. In the process, he was kept alive for more than a month when his outlook was clearly hopeless. At one point he asked whether I thought he was on his deathbed. When I said that he probably was, he replied, "That's what I think, too, and I wish they would just let me go." He complained to us on several occasions that too much was being done, that he just wanted to be left alone. In truth, we don't know what he said directly to his doctors, but we passed his concerns on to them, along with our own. We were assured that they were "doing everything possible" for our father. Everything possible included palliative surgery, blood transfusions, and intravenous feedings. Even his two physician sons, one of whom is on the staff of the same hospital, were unable, or too timid and conflicted, to influence the decision making so that he might be *allowed* to die sooner.

Having taken the earliest step—namely, an operation to try to remove the tumor—soon we were all swept up in a system in which it seemed only logical to take another step, and still another. For many years after my father's death I mulled over the irony that an intelligent, competent man, himself a physician, hospitalized in a major medical center, had absolutely no control over stopping useless treatment which everyone knew could not give him more time. His helplessness and frustration were shared by us all. It was never a question of assisted dying, only of having some degree of personal control. My father's death became the seed of my thinking on the entire subject.

It seems unfair that people who manage their own affairs successfully in life should be required to turn over so much of their death and dying to others. We direct the disposition of our belongings through wills and trusts, but except for the limited protection protection provided by "living wills," we have no such control over the conditions of our death, and the physicians who have this responsibility may be deaf to our entreaties and those of our families. Behind them stand tradition, a conservative profession, and the law. Regardless of a physician's personal compassion, helping people to die is risky in today's atmosphere. This atmosphere is changing, though, and one can already distinguish between the conservative views of medical societies—representing "the profession"—and those of practicing physicians who are concerned about the suffering of their patients. Many physicians have helped people to die, and many more would be willing to do so if it were legal.

This book is written for anyone who is concerned about how his or her own life may end and who wishes to avoid unnecessary suffering. Given a choice, most of us would like to live to old age, satisfied that we have accomplished what we could, and then to die peacefully, perhaps with enough warning to say our good-byes, but without undue suffering from prolonged illness. Old age, however, can be marred by severe disability, and death may not be kind or peaceful. Acute infections that killed swiftly and relatively painlessly fifty years ago have been replaced by organ failures and chronic diseases that take their victims slowly and sometimes very painfully. Through the passing of friends and relatives we have learned that there are good deaths and bad deaths, even horrible deaths.

The book is also meant for the caregivers who attend people who have fatal diseases. Family, physicians, nurses, and many others already participate in end-of-life decisions, but physicians will increasingly be asked to help implement those decisions through assisted dying. This will be a new and uncomfortable responsibility for these doctors. But the same modern medicine that has helped to provide us with great longevity shares responsibility for much of the distress experienced at the end of life. Medicine can add years to life but, because of legal restraints, cannot shorten it by even a few days. We are now beginning to be aware that this need not be the case. The very physicians who can help us to live so long could also help us to die more peacefully.

Finally, I hope that this book will be helpful for lawmakers as they listen to arguments for and against assisted dying. As proposals to liberalize their laws arise in state after state, responsible legislators will be expected to understand the issues well. Their job will be to respond to the needs of those who are suffering while protecting others from abuse. Well-reasoned laws can achieve both objectives, but the task of passing good legislation will be difficult.

The terminology associated with physician-assisted dying has acquired its own set of emotional meanings. One problem is the lack of an appropriate vocabulary for the emerging concepts. *Euthanasia,* the Greek word for "good death," was for centuries the right word. But it was totally debased in Nazi Germany, where mentally deficient children and adults were put to death involuntarily, in the name of eugenics and economy. In discussing physician-assisted dying, we have found no reasonable substitute for *euthanasia,* which still has that shadow hanging over it. *Suicide* is also heavily burdened, so much so that I shall devote an entire chapter to it. It is a word that is only now coming out of the closet, describing an act that still has an enormous stigma to overcome. A patient of mine who had breast cancer felt this way: "We need to rephrase the language of assisted dying to make it more understandable. *Suicide* is the wrong word, with its own meaning in our culture. I would like to hear *peace,* because pain is certainly a battle, even a war. You long for peace. We need to use more gentle language."

Even the courts have shown concern about the language used: "We are doubtful that deaths resulting from terminally ill patients taking medication prescribed by their doctors should be classified as 'suicide.' . . . We believe that there is a strong argument that a decision by a terminally ill patient to hasten by medical means a death that is already in process, should not be classified as suicide. Thus, notwithstanding the generally accepted use of the term 'physician-assisted suicide,' we have serious doubts that the state's interest in preventing suicide is even implicated in this case." The same court also said, "We believe that the broader terms—'the right to die,' 'controlling the time and manner of one's death,' and: 'hastening one's death'—more accurately describe the liberty interest at issue here."[1]

As public discussion of assisted dying has expanded, the language of the opposition has taken on harsh overtones. Terms such as *murder, self-murder* (suicide), *killing,* and *doctor-executioner* are used deliberately to inflame passions at the same time that they stifle reason.[2] The use of extravagant language discourages debate and polarizes the community at a time when the public would be better served by thoughtful consideration of all facets of such a complex issue. This is hardly new. Schopenhauer commented that "religious teachers are forced to base their condemnations of suicide on philosophical grounds of their own invention. These are so very bad that writers of this kind endeavor to make up for the weaknesses of their arguments by the strong terms in which they express their abhorrence of the practice."[3]

Opponents of physician-assisted dying knowingly use the word *killing* for its emotional impact. Their intent is to link the common concept of violent killing with the far less threatening concept of assisted dying. Killing implies the willful taking of the life of a person who does not wish to die. More philosophic and unassuming is "to die"—as in the war, or in an automobile accident—something that could happen to anyone. It is less personal and without malice. The agent of the death may not be known. This term is also applied at the opposite end of the violence spectrum—to natural death, as when a person dies in his sleep.

The crime of killing (or murder) requires a victim. The basis of our sympathy is that the victim's life is extinguished against his will. As a result, he is forcefully deprived of his entire future, of all the great and good things that life had in store for him.[4] But one can hardly speak of a person who is suffering and already dying, and who requests help to speed up the process, as a victim. He may be seen as a victim of his illness, but hardly of the physician who would help him die. Moreover, his future is not one to envy. Most if not all of the "great good that life had in store" is past. Not only may the future be distressingly short, but it is apt to be distressing in every other way as well. It is the desire to escape a few weeks of increasing suffering and total decline that leads to requests for help in dying. This should not be confused with a desire to be "killed" or "murdered." There is so obviously a difference between murder and helping a person die at his own request that gross attempts to blur the distinction are offensive. The public sees it, and ethicists and physicians see it too. Even the courts, with their rigid legal classifications, acknowledge the difference through their acquittals, if not their words.

What term then is best applied to the person who wishes to die and asks for help? The death is intended and expected, both by the person dying and by the person providing the help. Both also anticipate that the death will be accomplished in a gentle and humane fashion, not a violent one. The assistance is a compassionate response to an individual's considered wishes. The term that I will use is physician-assisted dying, rather than assisted suicide. *Dying* is a much more appropriate term than *suicide* for people who are already terminally ill. More accurately, assisted dying includes both assisted suicide, in which the patient must bring about his own death with materials provided by a physician, and euthanasia, in which the physician directly causes the death. Morally, they are quite similar activities, and eventually I think that both should be made legal. But there are also important differences, and in the immediate future the public, the medical profession, and our legal processes will be looking only at assisted suicide. So throughout this book, except where stated otherwise, I use *physician-assisted dying* only to mean assisted suicide.

In Chapter 1 I look at the dying process as it is encountered in painful and debilitating diseases, focusing on the needs of patients and their families, and on how these needs can best be met. More common than fear of death itself is fear of dying, particularly when the event may be prolonged, the expense considerable, and the person institutionalized, isolated, and beset with uncontrolled suffering. From the viewpoint of patients, good deaths are usually those that are quick, even unexpected, and relatively painless. Bad deaths are the opposite and are most frequently associated with cancer, pulmonary failure, kidney failure, AIDS, neurological diseases that produce severe weakness, and dementia. The special circumstances surrounding disability and eventual death from these diseases endows each of them with its own requirements with regard to assisted dying.

Any consideration of assisted dying, however, requires acceptance of the concept of rational suicide—namely, that there are circumstances when death is clearly preferable to continued suffering. The question of whether suicide is ever morally acceptable is really the heart of the controversy.

Chapter 2 reviews the history of our deeply ingrained religious, moral, and legal prohibitions against the act of suicide and presents the case for rational suicide as a necessary exception. Over the ages, suicide has been considered an unspeakable crime against God, nature, and society. It still remains largely unspeakable, but it is no longer a crime. It is illegal, however, for anyone to assist a person to die, regardless of the circumstances. The recent medical classification of suicide as an illness has brought about closer professional vigilance, but this is primarily in the area of prevention. Even in the face of terminal disease and intense suffering, the now legal act of taking one's own life is typically carried out in secret, and is all too often violent. Rational suicide, undertaken by a seriously ill person who wishes to end his suffering, is a new and challenging concept, particularly because it would so often require the help of a physician.

The key issue of Chapter 3 is the role of the physician at the end of life. Two medical responses to the needs of the terminally ill are evolving: better comfort care and assisted dying. Comfort care—the control of pain and suffering at the end of life—has received insufficient attention. People who have fatal illnesses should have all the support and relief that caring families, health professionals, and society can provide. Assisted dying should be seen as a last resort, an option to be considered when all other measures have failed or have been rejected. The hospice movement has enhanced our understanding of comfort care. But with increased understanding has come the realization that not all suffering can be controlled. Some people wish to be spared the exhaustion of waiting for the end and would forgo a few additional days of life in order to die more comfortably at home. Hospice cannot meet the needs of everyone. The current movement for assisted dying began in direct response to the requests of individual patients and has expanded to the level of public demand. Society's concern about unnecessary suffering at the end of life is reflected in recent polls, which show that about 65 percent of people in the United States favor legislation that would permit physician-assisted dying. Many feel that their own needs should be placed above those of their physicians or the medical profession. They feel that even the promise of help would increase their confidence in their physicians and would allow them to better enjoy their remaining days.

Physicians have always helped some patients to die. They are the obvious people to assume this responsibility when it can be done openly. The levels of physician assistance are 1) not starting or discontinuing treatment, 2) assisted suicide, and 3) euthanasia. These reflect very different levels of control and responsibility. The "rule of double effect" allows physicians to help significantly in the deaths of some patients by giving large doses of narcotics to relieve pain, with the knowledge that respiration will be suppressed and death may ensue. There are also many illnesses for which such medication is not appropriate.

In Chapter 4 I contrast a failed suicide attempt in the United States with an assisted death in Holland. A Dutch family whose experiences are described in detail accepted the ultimate outcome of the disease far in advance and participated in planning the death. Instead of secrecy there was strong mutual support and time to enjoy the final months together, free of fears about how it would all end. The act itself, carried out with a physician's assistance, was a gentle and painless sleep. It took place at home, the patient surrounded by the faces and voices of loved ones. They devoted time to reviewing life together, a life then slowly brought to a close in a spirit of love and appreciation. Dutch society differs from ours in several respects, but this social experiment is serving as a starting point for our own. Acceptance of planned death will require expanding the role of the physician at the end of life, with greater focus on the best interests of the patient.

Chapter 5 focuses on some of the physician's concerns about assisted dying, beyond individual religious and ethical beliefs. Personal concerns include fear of death and abhorrence of causing death, even to the point of seeing the loss of a patient as a personal failure. Although successful prosecution of a physician for assisting in death is rare, physicians are mindful that existing laws forbid such activity. Many attest that these laws are the primary reason, if not the only one, that they do not assist their dying patients more often. Doing less is safer.

A second source of concern is the medical profession, particularly its professional societies. The prototype, the American Medical Association, has been very conservative on most issues, and assisted dying is no exception. AMA leaders fear that such activity would result in a radically different role for the physician, damaging the physician-patient relationship and undermining trust in the profession.

Physicians must also face their own ethical dilemmas. Healing and helping to end life are contradictory goals. But relief of suffering and prolonging life are not always both possible. Assisting in a patient's death may be construed as doing harm in face of the strong professional admonition to do no harm. As a result, the compassionate physician must balance the request for deliverance from suffering against the many reasons not to provide help. It is hardly surprising that confusion and concerned ambivalence are common among physicians, many of whom are trying to formulate their own ethical standards in the face of considerable outside pressure but little real help. And all at a time of acknowledged moral and legal uncertainty.

Public concerns about assisted dying, discussed in Chapter 6, include the roles of various financial interests in prolonging or shortening life, the possibility of medical error, the potential for abuse, and the chance of a misstep onto a "slippery slope" leading to irreversible moral decay of our society. Abuse could come at the hands of family, custodians, or even physicians. The slippery slope could be a devaluation of life by individual physicians, the medical profession, even society as a whole. As a result, euthanasia could be legally extended beyond the limits of voluntary subjects to incompetents, and then still further to a spectrum of disadvantaged people: the poor, racial minorities, and the handicapped. These important concerns, which have become the cornerstones of most of the opposition to assisted dying, must be analyzed, understood, and addressed.

The differing views on assisted dying must eventually be assimilated into constructive laws that meet the needs of those immediately affected while protecting all others. In Chapter 7 I outline the precedent for such laws, the content of existing laws, and the legal steps by which similar laws might be established. In the background is a series of court decisions that have defined individual rights, decisions that could be extended to assisted dying. Intense legal review of the rights of individuals, under certain circumstances, to receive assistance in dying led two circuit courts of appeal to declare unconstitutional the statutes of twelve states forbidding such assistance. Reversal of these opinions by the U.S. Supreme Court indicates that the current court does not believe that choosing the time and circumstances of dying are legal rights protected by the Constitution. This decision means that no state *must* address this issue, but that any state *may* do so. Far from discouraging assisted dying, the Supreme Court decision is a signal that each state is free to meet the needs and desires of its own citizens. Oregon was the first state to pass a law permitting physician-assisted dying. For such laws to succeed they must include appropriate safeguards, but not so many restrictions as to make them unworkable. Several models are evolving through legislative attempts in different states. Some will succeed.

In the final chapter I summarize the major points for assisted dying and why I think the eventual passage of appropriate laws is certain to take place. In it I also review the options for private citizens, for the medical profession, and for state legislatures before such laws are passed. Physicians and society are already concerned about assisted dying, and doctors are under increasing pressure to accommodate new demands for more compassion and responsibility at the end of life, even though such accommodation is against the law in most states.

To better understand these issues I interviewed more than thirty patients who had serious illnesses and who would consider shortening their own lives, even if it required asking for help. I also talked to a similar number of physicians and a few nurses who care for such patients and would therefore be in a position to provide help, if it were legal. Although the numbers are too small to constitute a scientific study, the interviews were extensive and probing. The discussions were with real people, who had serious medical problems, and they helped me a great deal in my own thinking. Those patients who were not mine were asked by their own physicians if they would discuss assisted dying with me. I was amazed at how willing and even grateful many were to reveal their problems and concerns very openly. Many of the interviews were carried out in their homes. This preselection undoubtedly led to a biased sample. The physicians and nurses whom I interviewed were unscreened; I knew nothing of their views in advance. I have identified most of the people interviewed by their roles—a patient with colon cancer, a medical oncologist, a neurologist—rather than by using names or initials. I have attempted to maintain a gender balance in my writing by referring to all physicians as female and all patients as male. In addition, I speak of family in the broadest sense, extending it beyond spouses and blood relatives to the more inclusive "family of choice."

Four important social forces intersect in public consideration of assisted dying: rationality, morality, ethics, and the law. All appear as themes throughout this book. Each is subject to differing interpretations, and they also overlap and interact. More important, all of them are changing and are destined to undergo further change. A rational decision or action is one that is well thought out by a competent individual, for reasons that are understood and can be explained to others. To wish to die in order to be spared unendurable pain from illness is seen by many as perfectly rational. Morality is our common understanding of what is right or wrong, good or bad. It has evolved by common consent and governs much of human conduct. Although it is rooted deeply in tradition and is relatively stable, morality continues to evolve. Ethics, which began as the study of morality, generates theories to better understand and explain our moral thinking and to deal with necessary changes. Ethicists and philosophers have always been concerned about death and its reflection on the meaning of life. Now that this final event can be manipulated, with the possibility of extending or shortening life, the range of ethical thinking in this area is almost unlimited. Ethical approaches have been used both to support and to oppose assisted dying, so it is not surprising that they cannot lead us to any consensus or conclusion. They are arguments, not laws—analytical and persuasive, but limited. Finally, criminal law sets legal boundaries on permissible behavior, with tangible penalties for violations. Through such laws the state regulates the definition, trial, and punishment for criminal acts or omissions. The creation of laws by those holding elected office is basically a political process and therefore subject to public, private, and financial pressures. With its origins in moral and ethical thinking, the law is generally conservative and often slow to change. But the law is also born of reason and can respond to the pressure of rational argument.

For clarity I have included most of the points of view and arguments for and against assisted dying, reflecting the very different values of our society. As has been seen with many other sensitive issues, differences of opinion come into sharp focus and hyperbole abounds when it comes time to consider new laws. The process of creating social and legal change, however, begins and ends with the public. Appeals by individuals to their own physicians will overcome the resistance of the medical profession, and pressure by the public and physicians on state legislators will bring about the passage of more liberal laws. Major court decisions may hasten or retard the changes, but this is the process that must eventually take place. Quality of life to the last and control over the circumstances of dying are issues that touch everyone, and assisted dying will become legal and accepted when the public wants it to be. It is essential that the issues be understood, recognizing that today's needs are not necessarily met by yesterday's laws, that reason can counteract dogma, and that hypothetical fears of tomorrow's abuse and the slippery slope can be tested against today's reality in our own society.

Assisted dying is destined gradually to be accepted as an end-of-life option. The trend will begin with assisted suicide in a few states, then spread to other states as voters and legislators see that it is desirable and socially safe. After it becomes acceptable in many states, the courts may step back in to provide similar protection for people residing in more conservative parts of the country. Eventually assisted dying should be extended to include euthanasia for some people, and the range of underlying disorders should be extended to include neurological diseases that entail severe suffering but are not necessarily fatal, dementia, and even severe debility from old age. Assisted dying must be an option that can be requested by those who have lived with dignity and are determined to die the same way.

I find the world divides into those who've had the experience and those who are still fairly naive about what's involved in the dying process. Until you see someone you love really suffering, it is pretty abstract.
Wife of a cancer patient

I
The Needs of the Patient

My father, whom we have already met, was born in 1898, at a time when life expectancy in the United States was forty-seven years. He was born prematurely, and the family physician who delivered him warned his parents not to expect too much: his survival was unlikely. His incubator was a laundry basket behind the stove in the kitchen, the warmest place in the house. He survived and lived to eighty-nine, a satisfying old age even by today's standards. But the law of averages asserted itself, and his wife, my mother, died at the age of thirty-two, one week after the birth of her second child. The cause of her death was puerperal sepsis, or "childbed fever," a disease that took the lives of many young mothers until it could be treated by antibiotics. Her illness dispatched an otherwise healthy woman in just four days. My father's illness, superimposed on some of the physical infirmities of old age, lasted six months, of which more than one was spent in the hospital, supported by modern technology.

This vignette accurately illustrates what has taken place in medicine in this century, most of it in the last fifty years. From the point of view of personal suffering, deaths that were quick and relatively painless, usually the result of infection, have been all but eliminated. The tragedy of AIDS notwithstanding, far more people are now living longer, to the point where the average life expectancy of a child born today in the United States is almost eighty years. Most of this remarkable change can be attributed to better hygiene, control of infectious diseases, and the use of antibiotics. Now the spectrum of diseases that causes death has changed completely, to cancer, stroke, and heart disease. Added to these are a bewildering assortment of medical problems that gang up on the elderly and severely compromise their quality of life. Diabetes, hypertension, blindness, deafness, mental and neurological disintegration are just a few. The net result is that many deaths now are prolonged and sometimes very uncomfortable. So great are the numbers that almost everyone knows some friend or relative who had a "bad death."

The use of modern technology to support life is recent and interventional. Among the best-known examples are total artificial feeding through tubes or intravenously, dialysis, mechanical ventilation, and the use of artificial or transplanted organs. Collectively these represent the greatest advances of medicine since the advent of antibiotics. They also include supportive measures and procedures that can be carried past the point of futility and can extend life beyond the bounds of compassion. The problem that has evolved is obvious. Years ago people feared being snuffed out by disease too early in life. Now, in far greater numbers, they fear lingering deaths that may include years of being incapacitated and in nursing homes. Unfortunately, the worst fears of some are fully realized. Access to longevity, which few would refuse, forces us to accept the possibility that dying may be prolonged and profoundly uncomfortable. Public interest in assisted dying is centered on our fear of slow deaths associated with suffering that may be beyond our control, fear that is fueled by the sights and sounds of our hospitals, hospices, and nursing homes, a situation that is rapidly becoming more threatening to us as individuals and as a society. Today, however, we are beginning to realize that it does not have to be this way, that we can have longer, more fruitful lives and be spared the worst at the end.

Bad Deaths

In one sense, all deaths are bad; most of us would like to live as long as possible if we could do so on our own terms, free of the physical and mental failures of old age and of serious or prolonged suffering from disease. Because we have no control over any of these, we have every reason to look more closely at the actual circumstances of dying.

CANCER

It is obvious that some deaths entail far more suffering than others, and death from cancer is the most notorious. Cancer usually arises from a single cell that behaves and grows differently from its normal neighbor cells. Although most cells stop dividing and eventually die, the cancer cell continues to divide, developing a population in its own image that grows continuously. Within this new population, the normal controls exerted over cell division are eliminated, and the population becomes increasingly bizarre, a process known as tumor progression. The population expands at the expense of surrounding normal tissues and acquires the capacity to invade them. Thus a cancer of the rectum may eventually invade the wall of the pelvis or the bladder, making cure unlikely.

More lethal than local invasion is the capacity of many malignant tumors to metastasize or spread to more distant organs by the lymphatics or the bloodstream. In that case, the same cancer of the rectum may be caught in time to be totally removed locally, but not before its cells have spread to the liver, where eventually they can be fatal. Cancer respects few boundaries, and its behavior is truly anti-social. The unforgivable aspect of cancer is that it is our own cells, our own flesh that has turned against us and is bent on our destruction. Anger is understandable; in the words of a patient with colon cancer, "The greatest pain in cancer is psychological, the new thoughts that you get about yourself and the changes you find introduced into your life. Cancer is not only debilitating, it is also a demeaning disease. It says that your genetic structure is inferior, that your genes are just not up to it and your biological processes are rotten. So it is going to relieve you of the joy of living, because you don't deserve to live. You are a burden and you are going to suffer great pain."

The promise of medicine is frequently misunderstood, and medical treatment, with its very finite limits, often fails to live up to the hope that it generates. Unfortunately, the treatment of cancer causes its own share of distress. Treatment regimens that carry a 10 percent chance of success are enthusiastically promoted and are accepted by desperate patients. If the primary treatment fails, the secondary drugs may have only a 1–2 percent chance of success, but they too are offered and accepted. For the very few who benefit, many do not, and while failing to respond to the treatment, they suffer all of the injury and side effects without any gain. "Patients are often subjected to the most intensive protocols of chemotherapy, some of which require them to be taken to death's door in an attempt to eradicate their tumors. . . . Patients are pushed to the extremes of their endurance, and not always for reasons that include a careful appraisal of what is meant by the quality of life."[1]

Until the advent of the radical mastectomy in 1900, cancers were rarely cured. Moreover, death from this disease was usually slow, painful, and totally degrading. Pain was the hallmark of death from cancer and it remains so today, both in fact and in the mind of the public. The main difference is that palliative care of a person dying of cancer increasingly emphasizes the adequate use of narcotics to control pain. Physicians have varied and even wavered in their attention to this. Some fear that the risk of addiction requires that the doses of narcotics be kept as low as possible for as long as possible. Most, however, now understand that addiction is not really an issue for the patient who is dying. A more recent caution comes from the realization that large doses of narcotics can hasten death and thus perhaps be interpreted as illegal assistance in dying. Many physicians who are experienced with the treatment of cancer accept this risk. But despite the best efforts of hospitals and hospices, cancer remains an inglorious and frightening death.

AIDS

For more than a century, progress against infectious diseases and infections brought one major victory after another, beginning with vaccinations against smallpox and culminating with the use of antibiotics. This progress abruptly slowed fifteen years ago, not with the failure to control old diseases but with the advent of a new one that remains difficult to prevent or treat. Acquired immunodeficiency syndrome (AIDS) now affects millions of people and continues to spread uncontrolled in some parts of the world.

AIDS expresses itself as an assortment of disorders, all traceable to damage to the immune system by the human immunodeficiency virus (HIV). Unhealing skin sores and a rare tumor of the skin and subcutaneous tissues, called Kaposi's sarcoma, are the more visible manifestations. Beyond that, patients with AIDS suffer repeated infections. Eventually, they are gaunt, starved, and exhausted. The final causes of death are usually overwhelming infections, primarily pneumonia and meningitis. These infections are often opportunistic—caused by organisms that normally inhabit the body but are kept in check until the immune response is damaged by HIV and they have the opportunity to grow out of control.

The main toll from AIDS is among intravenous drug users and gay men. The two groups are similar in that they comprise mostly young people with lifestyles that may alienate them from their natural families. Beyond that, they are quite different. Intravenous drug abusers are more apt to be members of poor minorities, with limited incomes and weak social support systems that provide little help at the end of life. If their families do not stand beside them, they are apt to be quite alone. Gay men are often from the upper middle class, and better educated than members of the other risk group. A typical patient may have his own home or apartment and private health insurance and physicians. He often has a partner, a community of close friends, and extensive knowledge about AIDS, gleaned from experience within the group. Frequently, the result is a strong support system, including some friends who are willing to assist at the time of death. AIDS patients within the gay community have a very real interest in assisted dying, and, in some parts of the country, substantial experience.

Recently developed drugs can delay death from AIDS, but the price is high. The prolonged battle may result in blindness and dementia before surrender to a fatal infection. As one patient pointed out, AIDS has had a significant influence on attitudes toward assisted dying. "People are just living much longer than they had anticipated, and they are much sicker than they ever envisioned. You really don't know what it's going to be like until you're in the middle of it, and then what do you do?" In parts of California where AIDS has ravaged the homosexual community, a request to be put on a "morphine drip" is a request for assisted dying that is acknowledged by family, by friends, and particularly by physicians. The device is started with a high and sustained dose of morphine, usually at home, and a peaceful death is accomplished in a day or two. In a survey of physicians in the San Francisco area in 1995, 48 percent said that they would provide assisted suicide if asked by an AIDS patient, up from 28 percent in 1990, and 53 percent reported that they had done so at least once.[2]

The AIDS community on the West Coast has led the rest of the country in requesting and receiving assisted dying. As Susan Dunshee, counselor for AIDS patients and a member of the Seattle organization Compassion in Dying, attests,

> Suicide often comes up in discussions in AIDS support groups. Some people talk about it when they are first found to be HIV positive, thinking that they are already terminally ill. After a while, they get over this and realize that they can live comfortably for a long time, so that decisions about dying can be put off indefinitely. When they eventually do get sick, there is often much less panic than when they originally got the diagnosis. Some almost feel as if the other shoe has finally fallen and they can quit worrying. They turn their attention to how best to deal with their illness. As the disease progresses and quality of life diminishes, thoughts of how it all will end become much more important. They share a lot of common knowledge, including the names of physicians who have been understanding and sympathetic to their needs.

Physicians and money can be serious problems for AIDS patients. Some find helpful doctors; others do not. Many doctors refuse to care for them, and the cost of treatment can be tens of thousands of dollars per year.

NEUROLOGICAL DISEASES

Two neurological disorders, multiple sclerosis and amyotrophic lateral sclerosis (Lou Gehrig's disease), are associated with progressive muscular weakness. Multiple sclerosis, the more common disease, is characterized by attacks of weakness followed by stabilization or even remission, in cycles that may begin in the twenties and last for many years. Another form is steadily progressive, without remissions. The weakness affects any of several parts of the body, most notably the legs, face, eyes (leading to double vision), and the hands, where numbness and tingling can make it hard to hold objects.

There is often significant pain associated with the attacks. Eventually, the recurrences are closer and closer together until the progression is almost continuous. Death is usually from respiratory failure. Although very advanced multiple sclerosis causes a person to be bedridden, with almost total loss of mobility, mental competence is usually retained to the end. Because people with MS make remarkable adjustments, relatively few consider assisted dying until late in the disease.

Amyotrophic lateral sclerosis usually comes on between forty-five and fifty years of age and is characterized by weakness, muscle wasting, and cramps. The muscles melt away until a person is unable to move. Late problems include difficulty speaking and swallowing. There are no remissions, and about half the patients die within three years. Ten percent live about ten years, and a very few live twenty years or longer. Again, death is usually from respiratory failure. It is questionable whether the use of assisted ventilation is appropriate for people whose suffering is so great and prognosis is so poor. Patients with ALS are usually mentally competent to the end, with only 5 percent developing significant dementia.

Some patients with MS and particularly with ALS express interest in assisted dying. In the late phases of the disease, many say that if they had known what the symptoms were going to be, they would have taken their own lives. Later on, when they realize their predicament, they are unable to do so. Several such patients received help from Dr. Jack Kevorkian. The extreme suffering of one of these patients, shown on national television, produced a great deal of sympathy for their wishes to have earlier deaths and undoubtedly influenced the juries that have repeatedly acquitted Kevorkian.

The person with such severe weakness from a neurological disorder that he or she is unable to swallow raises an important issue about the type of assistance that can be provided. Laws permitting assisted suicide but prohibiting physician-induced euthanasia would appear to exclude such patients. But devices could certainly be developed that would be set up by the physician but activated by the patient—even by blinking an eye two or three times—so that technically the final step would be assisted suicide.

ORGAN FAILURE

Patients with pulmonary or renal failure can now be supported for indefinite lengths of time by appropriate equipment. Their lives can also be cut short by discontinuing the technical support—in about a week after ceasing dialysis or a few minutes after stopping respiratory support. Moreover, the mentally competent patient is now considered to have a legal right to have such artificial support discontinued, and the physician is expected to make the end of life comfortable. The nature of their support systems makes these patients unlikely candidates for assisted dying, but as we shall see, the legal acceptance of discontinuing treatment on request is a major argument in favor of assisted dying for patients with other illnesses.

DEMENTIA

Severe dementia is a horrible disability to contemplate, for the family who must witness it and for the thoughtful person who may anticipate it.[3] Strangely, total lack of memory or normal thought processes cause no suffering and produce very little problem for the patient at the time. The most common example of this disorder is Alzheimer's disease. A relative of mine developed this in her early sixties. The many activities that she enjoyed all ended in less than a year. The first clue that I had of any problem was after my cousin promised to leave the key to her apartment so that we could use it when she was away. She has a nice apartment in Washington, near a park, which she let us use from time to time when she was out of town. This time she forgot to leave the key and it took many calls to locate her and finally get permission to be let in. Usually when one is reminded of a promise made just a few days before, the person immediately remembers the conversation and apologizes that "it completely slipped my mind." This was not the case with my cousin. She could not recall promising anything three days before. Indeed, she didn't seem to remember that we had spoken at all.

Several similar episodes of "blanking out" happened, but it was about two years before the next symptom appeared—namely, inability to find certain words in conversation. This anomia, which might occur anywhere in a sentence, brought normal conversation to a stop while my cousin cast around for the right word, often substituting one or two synonyms as clues until someone supplied the correct term. In the space of a year this disability progressed from forgetting an occasional word to being able to express only a few words, and eventually no intelligible sounds at all. Her formerly animated expression became one of blankness, occasionally punctuated by confusion. Her once-fashionable clothes were now dowdy and dirty, and her apartment took on the unmistakable odor of incontinence.

She still lives in her apartment, with trained attendants and nurses around the clock. No one else goes in or out, except her son, who visits every two or three days and manages her affairs for her. She may live that way for a long time. Fortunately, she is wealthy— her nursing care alone costs $120,000 a year.

Alzheimer's disease is one of the more terrifying prospects faced by members of an aging population. It is estimated that 30 percent of people over the age of eighty will develop this problem.[4] The cost to families and society is already enormous and is destined to increase steadily. The dementia is progressive and irreversible, but the real tragedy is the slowness of the progression. The average duration of life after diagnosis is eight years, but with good care some can live more than twenty years.

It is small wonder that Alzheimer's disease is one of the great public fears and is already a controversial issue in many discussions of assisted dying. Responses from physicians interviewed for my study included their reactions to illnesses that they might someday have themselves, including Alzheimer's disease. Even the most conservative respondents, several of whom were totally opposed to the legalization of assisted dying, drew the line at Alzheimer's disease, saying that they would prefer to have earlier and more dignified deaths than put themselves and their families through the full range of horrors of this dementia.

A colleague of mine, Dr. Aaron Lerner, wrote poignantly of the death of his wife, Marguerite, from Alzheimer's disease.[5] Before her illness Marguerite was a successful physician and wrote children's books. She had a family and many activities and interests. She also was aware of her diagnosis before she lost the capacity to understand and talk about her illness. She made it clear that she did not want to go on living. For a year or two her most lucid hours were before daylight, and her husband taped some of her statements. "You need a new wife. This one is no good anymore. All I am is garbage. I belong in the garbage can. . . . I would rather be dead than what I am doing here, because I am not doing anything. . . . When can I be dead? Soon I hope. . . . I have lost a kingdom."

Marguerite's family promised her that she would never go to a nursing home, and she died at home a few years later. In an interview Dr. Lerner told me, "We had excellent care for her. Yet she suffered tremendously. The main difficulty was in seeing herself deteriorate. A proud person is put into an incredibly demeaning position. In addition, she would fall and break a bone in her hand or fall and have a facial laceration or cracked vertebra. Urinary tract infections were common. Even toward the end, when it appeared that she could no longer understand what was going on, tears would come to her eyes when I came home from work and said hello. I always felt that I let her down."

Many people want to be able to die before reaching the end stages of dementia. Arranging for such a death, though, poses very difficult ethical and legal problems. A few patients with Alzheimer's disease and a few more with Huntington's opt for preemptive suicide and take their own lives at the first signs of illness. Advance directives and instructions to those with durable powers of attorney may include requests not to treat acute infections that may provide "natural" deaths. But these requests are often voided by the family or simply overlooked by the nursing home.

In the future, when assisted dying is established for less complicated diseases, I think that it should be extended to formerly competent people with dementia. At the earliest signs of illness, or preferably before the onset at all, a person would have to write an advance directive and give durable powers of attorney to a family member or close friend, instructing that he be maintained throughout the early stages of the disease but that his life be ended by euthanasia to spare himself and his family the final stages. The turning point would be an arbitrary one, perhaps when he could no longer recognize members of his family. Such an arrangement would require agreement and cooperation between the patient, family, physician, and, if applicable, the nursing home. It would best be drawn up by an attorney who understood the situation. The patient would never know whether his plan was carried out. There would be no point in asking him, in the later phases of dementia, whether this was what he really wanted. The death previously requested would be outright euthanasia of a "person" who no longer understood anything.

The ethical issue, looked at from the outside, hinges on whether a person who is intellectually intact, the present self, can make a decision for the future demented self that is binding on those caring for him. Other ethicists look at the situation in retrospect, from the point of view of the patient with full-blown dementia, as the "now self" speaking of the "then self" as being the same person prior to illness.[6] The conflict is the same; the demented person may be living happily from day to day or, as we have seen, he may be tormented by the progression of the disease and the bleakness of the future. The demented person may be comfortable, carefree or even playful, but perhaps a year or two later may be physically restrained to a chair or bed, medicated for control, and covered with bed sores smeared with excrement.

The law professor and medical ethicist Ronald Dworkin wrote

eloquently on dignity and rights of the demented person: "A person's dignity is normally connected to his capacity for self-respect. Should we care about the dignity of a dementia patient if he himself has no sense of it? That seems to depend on whether his past dignity, as a competent person, is in some way still implicated."[7] Although the use of advance directives to request euthanasia at a time of future dementia is already being actively debated by medical ethicists, implementation is still far off. But I think that people who are farsighted enough to anticipate dementia will someday be given an opportunity to truncate it.

Daniel Callahan, an articulate opponent of physician-assisted dying, limits his assent in cases of dementia to nonintervention with life-extending technology.[8] "No one should have to live longer in the advanced stages of dementia than he would have in a pre-technological era," he writes. On the other hand, others even question the right of a demented patient to forgo the use of medical advances as requested in advance directives. "We do not advance people's autonomy by giving effect to choices that originate in insufficient or mistaken information. . . . Before implementing directives to hasten death in the event of dementia, we should require people to exhibit a reasonable understanding of the choices they are making."[9] I would submit that people who are aware and farsighted enough to prepare advance directives covering dementia usually know as much as or more than they want to know about the potential problem. A visit to a nursing home that has any significant number of demented patients can be easily arranged and will answer any remaining questions.

HUNTINGTON'S DISEASE

Another frightening illness that causes dementia is Huntington's disease.[10] It is inherited as a dominant gene, but symptoms begin only in the thirties and forties. Thus the victim usually has seen it first-hand through the death of one parent. The average lifespan after diagnosis can be ten or more years, and often much of the time is spent in a nursing home. In the early stages, the Huntington's disease patient is not only demented but shows a variety of awkward, purposeless movements that give the impression of drunkenness. Later these movements are so uncontrolled that it is necessary to be restrained to a bed or a chair. Still later, tube feeding is often required because of difficulty swallowing. The young person whose parent has Huntington's disease can now undergo genetic testing to determine whether he is going to get the disease or not. This can be done on infants or even in utero.

The clinical manifestations of Huntington's disease are so horrible and so drawn out that people at risk, or those who test genetically positive, often consider suicide, though few accomplish it. As the disease appears, insight and understanding about it disappear, so that a person who is determined to avoid the illness would have to take his life very early, at or before the time of the first symptoms. A good case could be made for a person with Huntington's disease, like the Alzheimer's patient, to prepare a comprehensive advance directive forbidding the use of any life-extending measures, including antibiotics; such patients may someday be able to arrange for assisted dying to be carried out at a late stage of the disease.

OLD AGE

Old age itself often seems to be a reason to want to die. Suicide is most common in elderly men. Assisted dying on request may someday be extended to people who are enduring the end stages of decrepit old age. By living longer we are exposed to a spectrum of diseases and to organ failures that cannot be avoided. The elderly have an advantage over demented people in that they can speak for themselves in the present tense. But the requirements for permissible assisted dying would have to be modified to accommodate people who might be suffering severely but might not necessarily be faced with imminent death.

Nursing homes are full of people "trapped in transit between retirement and death" because our health care system will not allow them to die, regardless of their expressed wishes.[11] Antibiotics that have been credited with saving so many lives can now be blamed for saving too many. The elderly person who wants to leave life behind should at least be allowed to do so, even though we are not yet prepared to help him. In the words of an eighty-three-year-old widow who took her own life, "In all other ways a law-abiding citizen, I am now obeying what I consider to be a higher law. The alternative would be unendurable. I simply haven't the courage to spend years dying by inches in a nursing home. I've earned the rest that only 'turning out the lights' will give."[12]

As the cost of maintaining an aging population increases, there will undoubtedly be more pressure to ration health care in some way. If the cost greatly exceeds the money available, health care will be treated as a "scarce commodity." This is already done in England, where waiting lists for procedures like hip replacements are so long that the elderly often die before they reach the top of the list. In the United States, livers for transplants are relatively scarce and changes in eligibility criteria for recipients are raising serious ethical issues. But before we contemplate rationing health care on the basis of age, consideration should be given to allowing the small number of elderly who are truly suffering and wish to have earlier and more comfortable deaths to do so.[13] This would be on the basis of personal rights rather than national economy because, as we shall see, the savings would be insignificant.

Bad deaths are too widely recognized by the public and acknowledged by the medical profession to be an arbitrary designation. The illnesses have in common frightening characteristics, including pain and suffering, loss of dignity and even an acceptable quality of life, and loss of autonomy and control. In small amounts these are the occasional setbacks of normal life. Bad deaths, though, are typically slow, with suffering that is drawn out and compounded to the point of being an unnecessary evil in its own right. The diseases are chronic and irreversible and can eventually be emotionally and financially exhausting. Nor do these enemies of acceptable life insinuate themselves one at a time. They attack en masse, eroding, degrading, and eventually overwhelming.

Pain and Suffering

Pain is part of human experience. We enter the world through the pain of childbirth and scream our objections with our first full breaths, our cries trumpets of victory to those who await us. The pain of childbirth is meaningful pain, limited in duration and rewarded at its conclusion. The pain of a broken bone is also meaningful. It demands protection from movement, the reward being complete mending. This pain inspired the ancients to use splints and the moderns to apply casts to immobilize broken limbs. Again, the pain is temporary and the gain is obvious. The meaningless pain of terminal disease, on the other hand, is permanent and destined to increase. It has no protective value, and it certainly is not blessed by any reward. The classic example is the pain felt with cancer. It is almost always the harbinger of worse things to come—including, eventually, death. Such pain has no redeeming or humanizing features. It is just there, open-ended, progressive and exhausting, a test of endurance for all concerned. "How much longer must this go on?" "Haven't I suffered enough?" These common questions imply the possibility of ending suffering at a time of one's own choosing.

All forms of suffering, including pain, are highly subjective. What is acceptable to one may be beyond the endurance of another. So wide is the range of our thresholds that the final evaluation of what is tolerable and what is not must rest primarily with the person who is suffering. Because there is no scale by which it can be measured, the definition and the limits of suffering cannot be readily imposed or interpreted by someone else.[14] For some, an earlier and more merciful death is the only answer to their suffering. A cancer patient of mine was explicit: "I am not looking for relief of my suffering. I am looking for it to end, totally and permanently."

With increasingly aggressive approaches, most pain can now

be controlled. Some can be relieved by new forms of narcotics, administered orally or through skin patches or by means of continuous infusion pumps. The use of other drugs to relieve anxiety and depression enables many people to endure their illnesses better. There are exceptions, however, where no amount of medication gives adequate pain control. In particular, cancer that invades or causes pressure on nerves may produce excruciating pain that is quite unresponsive to treatment. Typical responses of patients point to the drugs' ineffectiveness. "Who wants to suffer this kind of pain?" said a man whose prostate cancer had metastasized to the bone. "The medication puts me to sleep. As soon as I wake up there's the pain. If I can't live free of the pain, I'm not living at all, simply existing." A patient with cancer of the pancreas declared: "I would never have believed that there could be such pain. I am a different person. It's like having a new set of neurons implanted in my brain, each one producing as much pain as it can. And here I am enjoying the best of American medicine. I am ready to go now."

Moreover, pain of great intensity does not necessarily signify far advanced disease; it may have to be endured for a long time. Patient, family, and physician all suffer in this situation and share the hope that the end will come sooner rather than later. It is a time when the caring physician may truly feel that her hands are tied by today's legal constraints.

SUFFERING BEYOND PAIN

Suffering goes far beyond physical pain. Indeed, one large study showed that of people requesting assisted dying, fewer than 10 percent did so on the basis of pain alone.[15] Other symptoms that can be very distressing include breathlessness or a sense of suffocation, nausea, vomiting, inability to swallow or talk, urinary or fecal incontinence, diarrhea or constipation, coughing, sleeplessness, fatigue, weakness, and exhaustion from fighting disease. These symptoms tend to be cumulative and often overlap each other, making a miserable situation truly intolerable.

Personal losses that can cause intense suffering include loss of independence and dignity, as well as such basic abilities as walking, talking, or reading; strength, physical beauty, or sexual attractiveness; the ability to work and retain one's role as breadwinner or homemaker; and one's place in the community or family. A patient with lymphoma described his condition: "My major problem is total loss of strength. I'm as weak as a wet noodle. It's all I can do to get out of this chair and walk twenty feet to the bathroom and back again; then I'm literally exhausted, and it's not getting any better. The doctor assures me that a lot of symptoms can be overcome, but giving me strength is one thing he cannot do."

The person who is dying often finds his world getting smaller and smaller as his interests narrow down to those closest to him. These losses, existing and pending, are cumulative and can often cause someone to grieve in anticipation of his own death for the people and joys he must leave behind. The sense that the parting is definite and even imminent can cause great sadness and depression.

FEAR

Fear of what may lie ahead is a form of suffering in itself. Common sources of fear include failure to control existing symptoms, the advent of new symptoms and disabilities, and the possibility of becoming helpless and a burden on others. Many fear the institutions through which they may pass—hospital, nursing home, hospice. The extended twilight of a lingering death casts long shadows. We may fear loss of control over our lives, dirtiness and loss of dignity, abandonment by family, friends, or physician. We may fear loneliness, the unknown, or simply being at the mercy of technology. We may have financial concerns or regrets about the way we have lived or have not lived our lives. For some there is the raw fear of death itself, while others fear only that their dying may be truly painful. These fears are all part of being human; rare is the person who would not admit to experiencing many of them at some time in his life. Fear of what may lie ahead can underlie the desire for assisted dying even more than any suffering at the present time. For this reason alone, assurance that help and relief will be available if needed can be a comforting safety net that allows a person to tolerate suffering better and for a longer period.

Although fear can dominate the thoughts of anyone who is seriously ill, the roots of the fear extend much farther back in time. It is the possibility of having a horrible death that worries people who are perfectly well. These concerns, usually short of real fear, are sufficient to make a significant majority of our population feel that physician-assisted dying should be a legal option.

Dignity

Dignity is as easy to recognize as it is difficult to define. It centers around self-awareness and self-respect, a feeling of worth and pride, of knowing who we are, how we relate to others and to the world around us—"respecting the inherent value of our own lives."[16] It requires that we understand and accept ourselves, take pride in what we have done or are doing, and keep a sense of perspective about our past and our future.[17] Dignity usually includes having values that we know are important to ourselves and that frequently are recognized as good and worthy by others. It also includes a willingness to take responsibility for our actions and their consequences.

Each of us generates his own dignity throughout life, and we do not wish to see it soiled or smashed at the end. My father gradually lost the use of his legs while in his eighties. During one of my visits, when he could still get around with a walker, he excused himself to go to the bathroom. A few minutes later he called for help. He needed a clean pair of pants. "I wet myself. I didn't mean to. I couldn't help it." With a child's words, this proud, dignified, and totally responsible man began to cry, a sight his son had rarely seen before. A few minutes later, changed and comfortable, he used more characteristic language to express his frustration and damn his disabilities.

A dignified life deserves a dignified death. An appropriate death may be the kind of death that you or I would select for ourselves if we were given a choice. Personally, I hope to die peacefully at home, free of pain, and with family members nearby. But dignity at the end of life is not a given, and too often it seems not even to be a consideration. The person who is concerned about this must make his position very clear. One may reasonably ask, "Is the function of medicine to preserve biological life or to preserve the person as he defines himself?"[18] For some, loss of dignity can cause greater suffering than severe pain. Assurance by those around us, including family and physician, that the end will be neither protracted nor painful is recognition and appreciation of what we have been in life. It is this appreciation and this assurance that people are asking for when they request "death with dignity."

Quality of Life

Closely related to personal dignity is the quality of one's life. Both can be undermined by serious illness. Some feel that any emphasis on quality of life is hedonistic and a direct challenge to the religious concept of the sanctity of life, particularly at the end. With respect to assisted dying, Callahan speaks of the people's pursuit of "their private idiosyncratic view of the good life—even at the risk of harm to the common good," as if dying were a selfish pleasure voyage.[19] On the other hand, Helga Kuhse, director of the Center for Human Bioethics in Victoria, Australia, advocates an ethic based on quality of life, rather than unconditional sanctity, which "requires, unavoidably, the shouldering of moral responsibility—not only for allowing death to occur sooner than it otherwise would, but also for doing so on the basis of the quality or the kind of life in question."[20] Our tradition of religious freedom includes the right to pick and choose what aspects of religious teaching we wish to accept or reject, or even to reject religion altogether. The concept that life is given by God and can be taken away only at a time of his choosing

is not appropriate grounds for preventing those who do not share this view from doing what they think best. In our pluralistic society, such a restricted view should not have a place in formulating new laws.

A second related conflict exists between the concepts of quality and quantity of life. Here the medical profession is blamed for extending life beyond reasonable or desirable limits. The problem is that nobody would seriously want to be denied treatment or supportive care that could extend comfortable life, based on the possibility that his eventual death would be very uncomfortable. Indeed, even if one could know that suffering would be the price for a reasonable interval of satisfying life, most would accept it. People have every reason to want both longer lives and deaths that are free of unnecessary suffering. It is up to society, the medical profession, and legislators to make this possible.

Autonomy

If dignity and quality are important values right up to the end of life, autonomy is our way of protecting them. Personal autonomy is the liberty to make decisions for oneself, free from outside influence and constraints, and the capacity to act upon these decisions. Justice Benjamin Cardozo declared, "Every human being of adult years and sound mind has a right to determine what should be done with his own body."[21] The ultimate extension of autonomy is to control the time, place, and circumstances of dying. As such it is one of the central issues in any consideration of physician-assisted dying. A patient with liver cancer who was receiving chemotherapy in the hospital said, "If you commit suicide, you're not losing your autonomy, you're using it. You lose it when you get stuck in a hospital and they fill you full of all kinds of stuff that's not going to do any good anyway."

Patient autonomy is a concept that has been accepted only reluctantly by a traditional and paternalistic medical profession. Be-

fore the 1960s, the word *cancer* was rarely used in front of a patient. We had a variety of euphemisms, like "mitotic disease," by which we communicated with each other without using the dread word. With out knowing the nature of their diseases, patients could not possibly participate in any treatment decisions. At that time, few patients—much less their doctors—expected such participation.

As a resident at Massachusetts General Hospital in 1960, I spent several weeks assisting Dr. Claude Welch, one of Boston's great surgeons and one of my mentors. During that time I helped operate on a patient whom I knew well. She was the mother of one of my former classmates. This was a second operation on a woman who several years previously had had part of her colon removed for cancer. That much she knew. At the time of her second operation, when I was present, the tumor was found to have spread to her liver. Before leaving the hospital she told Dr. Welch that she *might* want to know "what the situation was," and she hoped that he would be able to tell her when she saw him in his office a few days later, if she asked. By today's standards, disclosure would be mandatory, but Dr. Welch, relying on the standards of that day, questioned whether he should tell her or not. When the time came she explained to him that she had many personal affairs that had to be settled and that she definitely wanted to know what her long-term outlook was. He gave her the information. She was grateful, even though it was bad news. In 1960, that was a new experience for us.

Openness in dealing with disease increased rapidly in the 1960s and 1970s. I associate the progress with the rise of the women's movement: women seemed to be more openly concerned than men about their health problems, and they demanded more information and eventually more control. Surgery for breast cancer is a case in point. The male-dominated specialty of surgery dealt with breast cancer differently from any other malignant disease. A woman with a breast lump, regardless of age, was hospitalized. She was given general anesthesia, and a biopsy was done. If it was negative, she woke up and was sent home. If it was positive, the anesthesia was sustained and she had a mastectomy. Nine out of ten biopsies were negative, but each of these women went to sleep not knowing whether she would wake up with her breast or not. No other cancer was treated that way. In almost all other cases the biopsy was a separate procedure from definitive surgery. Clearly, surgeons felt it was better that their female patients be spared what might be painful information and discussion. This unequal state of affairs came to an end when women began to insist upon more control over their medical treatment. A few years later an alternative form of treatment, radiation therapy, made it necessary to have a reasonable interval after the diagnosis of cancer in which to make a decision about the eventual treatment.

Another aspect of increased patient control is informed consent. Although the extent to which consent is truly "informed" is widely variable, the consent forms for new surgical procedures, for experimental or dangerous medical treatments, and for chemotherapy may run to several pages. The need to consent to medical or surgical procedures that carry significant risks has in itself made it mandatory that patients have some autonomy.

Orders not to resuscitate (DNR) and the use of advance directives and durable powers of attorney are all forms of autonomy that are initiated personally or delegated to a close family member. They are mostly negative—do not resuscitate, do not intubate—and are designed primarily to restrain the medical profession. They also extend our autonomy beyond the time when we can actively participate in any decision making. Medicine operates in a generally positive mode, so one usually does not have to request to have more done, except when disagreement arises over medical futility.[22] These negative forms of autonomy, which place great emphasis on protecting the right to be allowed to die, now include the right to discontinue life-sustaining support that is already in place, even if it requires the help of a physician to do so. This degree of autonomy is now well established, and the next phase of extending it even further is to be able to obtain help in dying when there is no support-ive technology in place.

THE UNKNOWN

Three objections to autonomy in end-of-life decisions are based on the unknown, the unknowable, and unequivocal mysticism. One argument is that causing death can never benefit a person because one must continue to exist in order to receive the benefit.[23] This metaphysical argument fails to take into consideration the fact that potentially beneficial treatment can completely fail. People who undergo high-risk surgery can die without realizing any benefit from the procedure, or, worse still, may survive so severely impaired that they would prefer to be dead. A parallel argument is that we should not have a choice between living and dying, because we do not know what it is like to be dead.[24] Although a life of suffering may be very uncomfortable, we cannot experience the alternative of no life at all. Barring a joyous afterlife, reports of which are infrequent and indirect at best, most of us have a very reasonable concept of what it's like to be dead. We do it all the time when we go to sleep. The difference is not in going to sleep but in failing to wake up, and frequently the fervent wish of the person who is dying is that sleep tonight will end it all, that there will be no tomorrow. On several occasions patients have said to me before surgery, "If you can't make me better, please just let me die on the table. I don't want to wake up." Our knowledge of what it is like to be dead is powerful enough to make it, under some circumstances, a very desirable state.

Finally, autonomy is widely accepted on the condition that it does not interfere with the similar autonomy of others. Some object to physician-assisted dying on the basis that our lives are part of a much larger complex, with mutual dependence on many others and even on our entire society.[25] This seems appropriate for team sports or military maneuvers that require integration and precision. But the number of people with whom we interact decreases as we get older or sicker, with fewer people depending on us to fulfill a role. As one's world narrows down to close family or companions, it seems inappropriate to try to enlarge it to a mystical universe of social interaction. Part of autonomy is being able to define our own universe, large or small.

Autonomy now allows competent people to accept or reject any and all forms of recommended treatment, regardless of potential value or risks. The physician is required to honor the patient's decision. A natural extension of this is to death itself, giving the individual the right to direct his life right up to and including the end. The corollary is that the physician should be able to honor her patient's wishes for help in dying if so requested. Indeed, the availability of physician-assisted dying creates another important option for the patient and clearly advances the level of personal control over dying. Recognizing the complexity of this issue and the wide range of our personal beliefs, a pluralistic society that claims to respect the rights of individuals should be tolerant in permitting seriously ill patients to choose freely how and when they will die.

Respect for patient autonomy has been one of the major changes in the practice of medicine in recent years, rapidly replacing professional authority and paternalism. A physician's refusal to share responsibility in decision making drives some people to seek more understanding doctors. The message that a new patient brought to me was quite clear: "He just wouldn't discuss it with me. He said this is what you should do and he let it go at that. When I talked to some friends and began to do a little reading, I realized it was not that simple, that I may have some choices. That is why I am here." Many medical decisions are now based on the perspective of the patient—it is his life and his suffering.

BEING IN CONTROL

For many, the concept of autonomy in a medical setting means having control over events at the end of life. The contested ground is over who should have this control. Opponents of assisted dying on religious grounds say that no one should be allowed to shorten his own life by so much as a day, though they allow physicians great latitude in extending life. The person who is dying may feel equally strongly that he would like to shorten his life by even as little as a day, just to be in control. This was expressed by a cancer patient who rejected the later phases of comfort care, including hospice. When he was awake he suffered severely. Morphine controlled his pain— but put him to sleep. He could see no reason for existing in this state until his disease finally overcame him. His family agreed when he said, "I want to die soon, regardless of whatever else you can do." Similarly, an AIDS patient noted: "It gives you some control again, at a point when you seem to have no control over anything." These and many other forces contribute to the current disagreement over assisted dying. The essence of the question is power.

As the opposing forces of patient autonomy and physician paternalism seek a new balance point, the important question with respect to assisted dying will be who should have the last word, who should be the gatekeeper—the patient who requests assistance, the physician who is asked to provide it, or the state that wishes to supervise it?[26] In the quest for a maximum level of self-determination, we should not lose sight of the fact that state approval of assisted dying will be coupled with requirements and restrictions. Until it is legalized, physician-assisted dying will be a very private matter between the patient who wants help and the physician who may be willing to provide it. The physician will wish to do so under circumstances that protect her own safety. Legalization will liberate patient and physician considerably, but then they will be expected to act within the rules established by the state. Guidelines already being considered include consultation with not one but two doctors and possibly even a mental health professional, along with many other requirements that will certainly be seen as infringing on autonomy. Ideally, the arrangement should be a private one between patient and physician, with as few outside limitations as possible. This will not be the case, however, under any legal structure now being considered. For absolute autonomy a person must take his own life without help. As soon as he wants assistance from a physician, he must expect to compromise and give up some element of control.

Although end-of-life decision making and activity will always require mutual understanding and cooperation between physicians and patients, the balance should and will continue to shift in favor of the patient. The strong trend is in the direction of greater autonomy, and this will continue because there are far more patients than physicians or lawmakers. Furthermore, every physician and lawmaker will someday be a patient. It is the patient's distress and impending death that require sympathy and even intervention. As requests become more numerous, physicians are going to find it difficult not to respond. Much legal and ethical thinking already stresses autonomy. Although the U.S. Supreme Court did not consider assisted dying to be a constitutionally protected right, many people feel that the ability to choose when and where we die is indeed a right, or at least a very basic personal interest. As that view gains acceptance, the autonomy of the individual will continue to expand.

FINANCES AND ALTRUISM

Whether out of love, loyalty, or a sense of obligation, the care that families provide can be expensive and exhausting. Recognizing this, many who are seriously ill are concerned about the emotional, physical, and financial strain that they may be causing their families. Protecting others is a time-honored motive for electing earlier death. As one cancer patient said to me, "I don't want to impoverish my children. They are just making ends meet as it is. I wouldn't want that on my conscience."

The personal costs of illness and care vary a great deal with circumstances but can be devastating for some patients and their families.[27] The majority of people have health insurance that covers illness of short and even intermediate duration. Medicare pays 80 percent of hospital costs for up to a hundred days for people over sixty-five. People who are wealthy can buttress this with insurance that goes much further. At the other end of the spectrum, people on welfare (Title 19) can get full coverage for unlimited lengths of time, providing them with quite good care. Of great political concern are the more than thirty million people in the United States who have little or no health insurance. This is a gap in our system that badly needs correcting. Embarrassing as the problem is, however, these are mostly younger people who are unlikely to have life-threatening diseases and therefore are outside of the patient group that we are primarily concerned with in this book.

The people who are most immediately concerned about the burden they may place upon their families and the health care system are those who require prolonged medical or custodial care to live with chronic diseases that will eventually be fatal. Alzheimer's patients serve as an example. Most patients with Alzheimer's disease are elderly, so Medicare will cover a hundred days of hospital or nursing home care. But the illness may last for years. Medicaid is available, but only after the savings and most of the income of husband and wife have been used up. They must provide as much care as they are financially able to before they can become eligible for Medicaid. The exact requirements are complicated and differ widely from one state to another, but a married patient in Connecticut is not eligible for Title 19 and Medicaid unless the couple's combined total assets are $1,600.00 or less. There is no legal way to protect the assets of one spouse, even in advance of the illness. With nursing homes costing from $35,000 to more than $80,000 per year and full-time care within the home even more, it is small wonder that the financial burden of an illness like Alzheimer's can be catastrophic. The entire savings of a married couple can easily be wiped out.

A patient of mine explained his concerns: "I worked until I was sixty-five and saved up a little money, which my wife and I are using to enjoy our retirement. We travel and do many other things that we had to put off until now. Our children are grown and independent, and we have no reason not to spend this money on ourselves. However, I want to spend it on things that we enjoy. Spending it to visit the children and grandchildren is one thing. Spending it to stare at four walls in a nursing home, unable to remember its name or address, is something else altogether. I have no intention of giving my money to a doctor who cannot help me, or a nursing home that I didn't choose and where I don't want to live."

Insurance to cover extended care is too expensive for most people. Grown children may feel obliged to contribute if they can afford to. (Unlike a spouse, they have no legal obligation to do so.) As the number of elderly in the population increases, the need for supervisory and custodial care is certain to become a major public financial issue, the cost of which may soon greatly outstrip the needs of the younger people who currently have no health insurance at all. Most Western countries that have comprehensive health care systems include long-term care in their coverage so that family assets do not have to be depleted. As the numbers increase in this country, so will the political pressure, to the point where we, too, may have to provide good long-term care at public expense.[28]

The question now is whether financial concerns should be included in considering an early death. The family may feel a strong obligation to do what it can, even though the cost may be ruinous. Some families are insulted by the implication that they are unable or unwilling to care for their elderly. The result is a strong sentiment in our culture that no one should decide that he has a duty to die for any reason, least of all for financial reasons. But what if the patient does not want to be a heavy financial burden on his family? As an alternative to keeping him in a nursing home for several years, he would prefer that his children have their own home, or that his grandchildren go to college. With a nursing home costing as much as $80,000 a year, these are legitimate concerns, and I think that a competent person has a right to take them openly into consideration. I do not think that it is necessarily wrong to wish to die for altruistic reasons. There should be other valid reasons too, but the burdens that chronic illness place on some families can be inescapable and ruinous. This view was shared by the U.S. Court of Appeals for the Ninth Circuit: "We are reluctant to say that, in a society in which the costs of protracted health care can be so exorbitant, it is improper for competent, terminally ill adults to take the economic welfare of their families and loved ones into consideration."[29]

Having looked at many reasons why a person who is seriously ill might wish to shorten his life, we must now recognize the fact that such an act, with or without help, is essentially suicide. Is it ever acceptable?

People who insist that life must always be better than death often sound as if they are choosing eternal life in contrast to eternal death, when the fact is that they have no choice in the matter; it is death now, or death later. Once this fact is fully grasped it is possible for the question to arise as to whether death now would not be preferable. Death taken in one's own time, and with a sense of purpose, may in fact be far more bearable than the process of waiting to be arbitrarily extinguished.
Mary R. Barrington

2 Rational Suicide: The Core of the Controversy

The central issue in physician-assisted dying is the concept of rational suicide. The basic definition of suicide includes the intended death of oneself, carried out by oneself, under circumstances free from outside coercion. The question now is whether there are any circumstances when such an act is reasonable, rational, and morally acceptable. Traditional medical and psychiatric thinking considers all suicides to be the product of disturbed mentation, usually depression, and therefore irrational. But the concept of rational suicide, widely held in ancient Greece, is reawakening in our culture. Although it will always apply to only a small minority of all deaths, this concept is rapidly gaining acceptance among patients with terminal illnesses and the physicians who care for them, as well as with medical ethicists and others who concern themselves with end-of-life decisions. The dilemma of a person who is painfully and terminally ill, faced with our current restrictions on suicide, has made it necessary to reevaluate our attitudes toward suicide, as has the plight of those being kept alive, after life has lost all value or meaning, with extreme application of modern technology. These issues underlie the concept of rational suicide. There are indeed people whose dying is so prolonged and whose suffering is so intense that their desire for an earlier and more comfortable death is easily understood by and acceptable to most people.

Many people with fatal or progressive and severely debilitating diseases reach the point where their suffering seems needless and cruel and where they would prefer an earlier and more comfortable death to living out the natural course of their illness. They have well-thought-out reasons to wish to end their lives sooner rather than later. Such a person has a legal and moral right to refuse treatment and even elementary maintenance care. Beyond that, should he have the means at hand, he may take his own life. Legal for several years, the morality of this act is gaining acceptance on the basis that it can be an entirely reasonable and rational wish.

A patient with colon cancer stated, "How and when I'm going to die should be my decision. It would give me great comfort and peace to know that nothing on earth is going to cause me to suffer pain or a nasty death, being totally dependent. There's my escape, right in the palm of my hand. I'd like that. It would give me control over my own life and body that I don't have now, but which I think I'm entitled to." Others have expressed similar thoughts. According to one author on the subject, "It is rationally justified to kill oneself when a reasonable appraisal of the situation reveals that one is really better off dead."[1] Another wrote: "As soon as it is clear, beyond reasonable doubt, not only that death is now preferable to life but also that it will be every day from now until the end, the rational thing to do is to act promptly."[2]

Rational suicide, with or without assistance, has two major foundations: the desire to avoid unnecessary suffering and the desire to exercise one's autonomy and self-determination. Even though these may not be explicitly stated, the first is an essential reason for wishing to have an earlier and more comfortable death, and the second provides the impetus for actually doing it or asking for help. It should be noted that the criteria for rational suicide apply equally to all forms of assisted dying, for all such actions are initiated by the patient and are similar in many ways. The benefits of an earlier death, in the eyes of the patient himself, should exceed or at least be equal to the costs that will be exacted. In general, rational acts produce well-being and reduce harm. This is the essence of electing earlier death over prolonged suffering. The criteria for rationality in the desire to die fall into three categories: the nature of suffering that is to be avoided, the decision-making process, and the decision-making capacity of the individual. We must look at these criteria mostly from the point of view of an objective outsider, because most patients consider themselves to be rational, whether someone else would or not.

Rationality

We have examined many forms of suffering that a person who is seriously ill might wish to avoid. They all result from having a hopeless condition, for which improvement or cure cannot be expected, and they include terminal illness, pain and suffering that are intractable and unbearable, or a progressive debilitating condition. Any of these could reduce the quality of life to an unacceptable level. Imminent death is not a requirement for a rational wish to die. Although their suffering may be great, I do not include people whose reasons for wishing to die are due to primary mental illness or to pain that is purely psychological in origin.

Several components should be included in a sound and rational decision-making process:

1. One should have the ability to understand and assess the illness itself as the cause of the suffering that is to be ended. Closely related is the

ability to understand and weigh all of the alternatives to earlier death, including further treatment, comfort care, or hospice.

2. A rational decision should involve some understanding of the impact an elective, earlier death would have on family and close friends.

3. The decision should not be an impulsive one, but should be considered carefully over a period of time.

4. Ideally, the rationality of a decision to die should be tested on an objective listener of one's own choosing. As will be seen, however, until rational suicide and assisted dying are more widely accepted, such a consultation is apt to be avoided by the patient who is truly rational and understands the risks.

5. A decision to end one's life should be compatible with other personal beliefs and values. Religious beliefs are the most obvious, but even strongly held values are sometimes discarded in favor of the desire for relief and autonomy when the stress is severe.

The rationality of an act is often more easily defined by common usage, even through examples, than it is in concrete terms. Because end-of-life decisions can be nonrational, irrational, or rational, we must explore these distinctions. A Jehovah's Witness may refuse blood transfusions, even when they are necessary for survival, because of nonrational religious beliefs. Similarly, a person of strong faith might feel that he has to endure life to its natural end, regardless of suffering. This would also be a nonrational, religious issue; he must do it. Nonrational acts are borne of belief systems, rather than evolving from the world of common experience. They are "matters of faith rather than reason" but are widely recognized in our society as acceptable exceptions to the rational-irrational diathesis.[3]

The teenager who despairs over a dissolved love affair may consider his options very carefully and conclude that death is the only way to end his misery. Society, however, considers his suicide to be a completely irrational act and feels justified in doing whatever possible to intervene. It knows that he is too young and distraught to understand that he will get over the feeling of despair at his loss and probably live a normal and even happy life, if he can be persuaded not to take such an irreversible step. The admonition of Edwin Shneidman, a scholar of suicidal behavior, applies here: "It is not a thing to do while one is not in one's best mind. Never kill yourself when you are suicidal."[4] Realizing that the entire community would reject his plan, the teenager cannot discuss it or in any way test its "rationality" on other people. A survivor of a leap from the Golden Gate Bridge is said to have defined suicide as a permanent solution to a temporary problem. Although the young person who is temporarily distraught has a legal right to take his own life, society feels otherwise, and most agree that such untimely deaths should be prevented whenever possible. In this sense, the will of society is allowed to override the autonomy of the individual for his own good, precisely because his reasons for wanting to die are probably temporary and are generally considered to be inadequate.

The seriously ill person who anticipates a bad death but wishes to avoid unnecessary suffering has a completely different problem, and consideration of an earlier death may be totally rational. He may ponder his position very carefully, weighing a few more days or weeks of life against relief from his suffering. He knows that it is not a temporary situation. The illness will get worse, not better, and death is impending, if not imminent. As the end of life draws close, time does become a central issue. Must he wait passively, as some would require, for his disease to overwhelm his body and exhaust his resources, finally producing a living corpse whose meaningful life ended weeks ago? Or should he be free to choose his own hour of departure, to meet his own needs and desires, with the elements of personality and personhood intact and a mind still able to make a final and most important decision, the decision to die on his own terms, when he may indeed be in his "best mind." He may have no strong religious or moral reservations, and no personal or family obligations that will be satisfied by a few additional weeks of life. Indeed, under optimal circumstances, if physician-aided dying were legal, it could be discussed with others, including family members who have the greatest concern and the physician who might be asked to help. The dying person might also realize that his wish for a timely death is rational in the eyes of many people, that a significant majority feel that there are medical circumstances when an earlier death would be acceptable and should be legal. Few would deny a dying person the right to continue his existence, even with futile medical support, in the irrational hope that a cure is just around the corner. Why, then, should we deny an earlier death to someone who rationally understands and accepts the hopelessness of his situation?

A more complex example is the person who has a recognized depressive disorder but who also has a devastating terminal disease. Such a person might present his case very rationally and be legally competent to make most medical decisions, most of the time. Should this include rational suicide? In this borderline case I can see where compassion for suffering could outweigh concerns about questionable competence or rationality. A still more difficult example is the person whose only problem is a persistent serious depressive disorder that does not respond to treatment. Severe depression has been accepted as a justifiable reason for assisted dying in Holland, but I do not believe enough is known about this type of disability to consider its inclusion in the United States. People with severe depression are not dying. Indeed they can live normal life spans. More important, remarkable new drugs have become available to treat depression, and more can be expected. The result is that people who are depressed but not dying or suffering from irreversible disorders may very well benefit by waiting for effective treatment to be developed.

There are some general but simplistic concepts of rationality that do not apply to rational suicide or assisted dying. Rationality is often construed as being based on common sense and social norms. In a sphere that is so new and controversial, judgment by these criteria will hardly be possible. Similarly, rational acts are thought by some to be those that are convincingly rational to others. Again, the listener may agree or may have entirely different thoughts on the subject. Even mental health professionals can have strong prejudices in this area, casting doubt on their other qualifications as judges of rationality. Instead, the rationality of an individual must be looked at very objectively, based on his own understanding of his own situation.

A rational decision of such magnitude requires that a person has acceptable decision-making capacity. This evaluation includes the most contentious points in any consideration of rational suicide or assisted dying, if only because it is much more difficult to verify than are suffering and other components of the decision-making process.

1. The decision should be an autonomous one, a personal choice made in the absence of outside pressure.
2. The individual should be mentally competent to make a life-and-death decision.
3. The decision should be made in the absence of treatable clinical depression.

COMPETENCE

Competence is a legal concept, but one that often requires medical evaluation. Most physicians feel that they can judge the competence of their patients to make medical decisions, even those involving life and death. Psychiatric evaluation is rarely requested. In emergencies, major medical decisions are often made by patients who are presumed to be competent, even under the most stressful conditions. These include the competence to accept or refuse potentially life-saving but risky surgery. A competent person is expected to demonstrate rational qualities of decision making, including understanding the disease, the options, and the consequences of treatment or lack of treatment. He should be able to express his own choice clearly, though he need not defend it. Finally, he should be able to communicate this intelligently to his doctor. A psychiatrist would almost certainly go beyond this and attempt to evaluate the patient's general mental status and level of function.[5] An attorney for Yale–New Haven Hospital explained the hospital's legal position: "Competence is a decision-specific process. A person might be judged incompetent on the basis that he cannot remember the year or balance his checkbook. However, if that person understands the consequences of the medical decision that he is making—that is, he understands that he is going to die and it seems to you that he understands what death means—then it really doesn't matter whether he's oriented to the month or year."

A person who has no psychiatric illness but is for any reason mentally deficient may be deemed incompetent to make medical decisions. Conversely, a person with an underlying primary psychiatric depression, but who also happens to have a terminal illness, may be perfectly competent to give rational reasons for wanting to die. Obviously, his background depression would cast doubt on his current reasoning.

The Dutch psychologist A. Kerkhof sees competence as a relative value, particularly in making major decisions.[6] He draws an analogy between end-of-life decisions and other major decisions like marriage and divorce. Although marriage and divorce are not so final, all three situations involve unknown factors that one cannot foresee or comprehend. The future can be looked at hopefully but never incontestably, and decisions frequently involve the lives of others. In marriage and divorce, people are encouraged to examine their thinking but are given the right to choose, however good or bad their choice may seem to be.

Some claim that rational thinking is not possible when a person is suffering from intense pain, that the pain itself is a form of coercion. It has been argued that pain and the side effects of narcotics are very apt to render a patient incompetent.[7] In more general terms, Freud questioned the rationality of suicide, saying that "it is indeed impossible to imagine our own death—in the unconscious everyone is convinced of his own immortality."[8] The problem here is that the severely ill person who wishes to die is not speaking from his unconscious but from the conscious level, at which he is feeling his pain and suffering. Moreover, the reality of progressive disease may overcome any illusions of immortality, either conscious or unconscious. Finally, it should be noted that Freud obtained help in taking his own life when he was suffering from advanced cancer.

The depression-incompetence-suicide dogma is now being challenged by concern for autonomy and personal choice in matters surrounding the end of life, particularly in the presence of severely incapacitating or terminal illness. A person is presumed to be competent and able to make all medical decisions until proven otherwise. This is already widely accepted for patients who refuse life-prolonging treatment. The competence of a person who requests that life-supporting technology be discontinued is rarely questioned, nor is his legal right to have his request fulfilled. The extension of this concept to suicide and physician-assisted dying is an important and central issue—that is, the wish to die should not in itself be considered to be an indication of incompetence.

Why has competence suddenly become important? Perhaps society and the medical profession find rational suicide and physician-assisted dying so hard to accommodate that any excuse is useful, even if it is not consistent with other accepted actions. The law and the medical profession no longer seriously question the competence of a person who refuses treatment, even when the results would be predictably fatal. When a patient has a newly diagnosed cancer, the physician has an obligation to provide all the facts about the disease and to try to persuade the patient to choose a "wise" course. But when all fails, competency is almost always assumed and the refusal accepted. Psychiatric evaluation is usually turned down, if suggested at all. Much more common is the decision to discontinue treatment because the long-term gains do not justify the discomfort of further therapy of a disease that is obviously progressing. Many cancer patients eventually reach this point. Again, the competence of these patients to make such decisions is not questioned, even though life may be significantly shortened.

Finally, in any interactive relationship, such as that between physician and patient, the role of the physician must be looked at critically too. There is obviously danger that the patient's values may be disregarded if they differ from those of the physician. A revealing situation was reported in which two psychiatrists disagreed in court about the competence of a patient who wished to die.[9] The psychiatrist who thought the patient should be considered incompetent explained that "it comes down to a philosophical difference. I hope there is no psychiatric argument in this case. It is the right of a patient to decide he wants to die, but I spend all my life trying to keep people alive so I take quite a different view."

In the context of such restrictive thinking, all roads lead to incompetence. This is very unfair to the patient who knows who he is in life and where he is in respect to his disease, and who has given serious thought to his eventual death. Limits have indeed been placed upon him. The disease, with its pain and suffering, is fatal and will not go away. Death may still be feared, but it is no longer unexpected. It would be unusual for a person who is slowly and painfully dying, and who is fully aware of his plight, not to experience at some time elements of sadness and depression, sadness over his impending losses and depression over his relentless disease. The expressed wish to die is looked upon by some as in itself diagnostic of mental incompetence. If suffering and pain are forms of coercion or cause incompetence, they will continue to do so to the very end. Narcotics may help, but they do cloud the senses. As the dose increases, contact with everything that matters decreases. And this, too, continues to the bitter end. One can have drugs and no pain, or pain but no drugs. The physician who "knows best" may be so preoccupied with her own dark angel as to be quite deaf to the entreaties of her dying patient. The patient must live with all of these limitations. They cannot be avoided. It can be argued that if by all other criteria a person is competent, but he wishes to die, he is really demonstrating his competence rather than his incompetence in asking that his autonomy be respected. The medical-legal evaluation of one's competence is made by others, but the criteria should be the same as would be applied to any other serious medical decision, including refusal of treatment.

Unless one accepts the assumption that anyone who wants to die is by definition incompetent, most patients who have serious illnesses and express such wishes are perfectly competent. Fortunately, this restrictive definition is not widely accepted. Psychiatric consultation is rarely sought to determine competence in such patients and may not be preferable to evaluation by the primary physician.[10] In the many patients interviewed in this study, competence by the usual criteria was never in doubt. They would have been insulted or amused if their competence for decision making was even questioned. Among them, however, were many who wanted their suffering to end sooner rather than later.

DEPRESSION

Depression is a major diagnostic issue that is often placed before psychologists and psychiatrists. It is also central in the controversy surrounding rational suicide. The similarity between primary or clinical depression and reactive depression that is secondary to serious illness is receiving increasing attention, particularly by psychologists and psychiatrists who routinely deal with seriously ill and dying patients.[11] The following outline is adapted from George M. Burnell, M.D., and a discussion with James Ciarcia, M.D.[12] The physical signs and symptoms of depression are very much the same, regardless of whether it is a clinical depression or is secondary to debilitating or fatal illness. Insomnia, fatigue, loss of energy, poor appetite, and weight loss are commonly seen in advanced disease as well as in clinical depression and do not help to distinguish between the two. Similarly, feelings of hopelessness may be nothing more than a realistic self-appraisal for the dying patient.

Beyond these common characteristics there are some significant differences between the suicidal person who has clinical depression and the seriously ill patient who wishes to die. The background of the person with clinical depression is apt to include a
history of previous episodes of depression, which may even have required treatment; often there is a personal or family history of depression and even suicide attempts. The depression may be precipi-
tated by a major loss, such as a death, loss of job, or loss of a partner.
The person is often withdrawn, with a history of poor relationships
and little concern for others. At a cognitive level are low self-esteem
and expressions of worthlessness, guilt, shame, and a pessimistic
outlook about life in general. There is also apt to be a marked degree of anhedonia—the person gets no pleasure or enjoyment in
doing or anticipating anything. The death wishes are often self-
destructive and violent, tinged with anger and wishes for revenge.
The thoughts and reasons for suicide are self-centered, with anger
directed against oneself for personal inadequacies and rebuke by a
world that is not understanding. Obviously, many such people also
have serious illnesses that make their private problems worse.
Strangely, episodes of clinical depression are usually self-limiting.
Given some time, they resolve spontaneously. When there is a single obvious cause, the loss of a spouse or dissolution of an important relationship, recovery is usually permanent. In bipolar depression the patient often realizes from experience that he will recover,
although he may not think that he will recover this time. He also realizes that the cycle will repeat itself.

By contrast, the wish to die expressed by the seriously ill patient who has no associated mental disorder is directly related to the
illness itself. This "reactive" depression starts with the illness and is
built around it, an illness that is known to be fatal or at least progressive and incurable. The patient often has to deal with moderate
or severe pain, extended treatment that may be quite incapacitating,
and a genuinely grim long-term outlook. The result is often exhaustion from the disease process and its treatment. There is usually no

family history or personal history of depression or previous suicide attempts. Indeed, there are usually close and continuous family and personal ties, including real concern about what the death will mean to others. Rather than being self-centered, the death may be seen as a form of altruism, to avoid being a burden on others, sparing them the exhaustion of extended care and personal and financial stress of a prolonged illness. The background of the patient is often that of an active person who was used to taking responsibility. Any significant previous losses were adequately accepted and are not central to the current thinking. Instead, the blame is directed toward the disease itself. The conditions caused by the disease are demeaning and intolerable, and the patient is concerned about loss of dignity and self-respect. He often has a well-thought-out personal philosophy about life and the meaning of his own death, possibly even having to rationalize the current desire for death against a moral and religious background that forbids such activity. He does not believe that his decision is immoral or wrong. At a cognitive level this patient feels no guilt or regrets about his past life but rather expresses pride in his accomplishments and in having been a "good person."

Even when there is very little pleasure to be had, the dying patient still enjoys special people and events and can anticipate good things. He may have some limited goals and purposes for his remaining life, such as arranging his finances. His sense of humor is apt to be retained, often as black humor directed at himself, the physicians, or the illness, but intended and recognized as humor. An AIDS patient described his interaction with his physician as follows:

> He's very honest and, most importantly for me personally, he's got a twisted sense of humor, just like mine. He called about a week ago saying he needed to repeat my blood work because he didn't like that last set of figures. When I asked what they said, he replied, "Well, according to the numbers you're dead. I'm going to have to draw it again because nobody else will touch you in that condition." I found that very funny, coming

from a doctor. We understand each other and he knows that I'll laugh. If he meant it, he would never say it. He can also get very serious and candid when he needs to be and that's why I trust him. I have not discussed dying with him yet. But I sense that it is not going to be difficult and that he will help if I ask.

Finally, the dying patient considers the disease to be a violation of an otherwise normal life and views death as a release from suffering. He would truly prefer to live if he could live normally, but that being impossible, he would prefer death over his current condition. Similarly, being neither angry nor self-destructive, he would prefer a gentle rather than a violent death, a death provided with kindness and love and with the approval of close family members. George Valliant pointed out that hopelessness is a common denominator in many suicides but that we know very little about what hope really is, how it works, or why it is so important.[13] The reactive depression that is associated with terminal illness is tinged with sadness in departing what was previously a happy life and at leaving behind truly beloved family and friends. According to Yeates Conwell and Eric Caine, "The distinction between the depressed mood or sadness that develops as a natural response to serious illness and the clinical depression syndrome for which treatment is warranted is a subtle one that should be made by a physician."[14] As Kerkhof described it: "It is not clinical or mental or psychotic depression. It is a natural form of depression, part of the process of adapting to a terrible situation."[15] Even Herbert Hendin, who strongly opposes assisted dying, said, "The person facing imminent death who is in intolerable pain and arranges to end his life may be a suicide in the dictionary definition of the term, but not in the psychological sense."[16]

Background

The background to our current thinking about rational suicide is important to understand because every step has made a lasting contribution to the current debate. As Joseph Fletcher points out, "The full circle is being drawn. In classical time, suicide was a tragic option, for human dignity's sake. Then for centuries it was a sin. Then it became a crime. Then a sickness. Soon it will become a choice again."[17] We now turn to the history of social, religious, legal, and medical attitudes that underlie our current thinking about suicide. Although these attitudes evolved in sequence over many centuries, they are all still present and influential today. Suicide is now considered to be a medical problem, but the church and state have maintained strong interests in it.

THE ANCIENTS

Suicide was widely accepted and practiced in ancient times, certainly in Greece and Rome.[18] Sophocles, Zeno, Seneca, and Pliny all wrote approvingly of suicide and even encouraged it. It was considered a rational response not only to health problems but to all problems in life that seemed overwhelming. The Romans extended this philosophy and condoned suicide to preserve honor, to avoid capture or imprisonment, as an expression of devotion to a loved one who had died, and for patriotic and political reasons. The first-century A.D. Stoic philosopher Seneca is widely quoted on suicide: "Against all the injuries of life I have the refuge of death. If I can choose between a death of torture and one that is simple and easy, why should I not select the latter? As I choose the ship in which I sail and the house which I shall inhabit, so I will choose the death by which I leave life. The wise man will live as long as he ought, but not as long as he can."[19]

Even the philosophers who opposed suicide made exceptions for people who were incurably ill and suffering. These exceptions were almost universally accepted and are the forerunners of our current thinking about rational suicide. It is also important to note that even in the fifth century B.C., when Hippocrates began his practice, most of the "medical profession," such as it was, was completely free to aid the person who wished to die. Indeed, this was probably an important role for the ancient physician. The methods available included poisons and cutting open of veins to allow fatal hemorrhage. The liberal thinking of the Stoic physicians gained ascendancy at the time of the Roman conquest of Greece and was almost universally accepted during the first two centuries A.D. Eventually, the value of human life was trivialized in the Roman Empire. Public torture and executions were extended to killing for sport and entertainment. People even volunteered for such executions in order to gain financial rewards for their families. Not until the rise of Christianity was suicide stigmatized.

RELIGION

Expanding on the remnants of conservative Greek thinking and the established doctrine of Judaism, and perhaps in reaction to the excesses of the Roman Empire, Christian doctrine forbade all killing, including both suicide and abortion. The earliest days of the new religion saw constant conflict with the Roman state, often resulting in martyrdom. To condone this type of "suicidal" behavior, the Church decreed that martyrs had instant and direct access to heaven. Religious fervor and the desire to obtain a beautiful afterlife led to an increase in the number of martyrs, and possibly even volunteers for martyrdom. This was brought to a stop in the fifth century A.D. by St. Augustine, who cited the commandment "Thou shall not kill" as the basis for prohibiting any taking of human life. Political reality, however, required exceptions to this rule, for war, capital punishment, and self-defense. Clearly, Christ's personal pacifism and admonition to "turn the other cheek" was not functional for a religion that wanted to establish itself in the real world.

In the early days of Christianity the penalty for suicide was relatively mild, a delay for the damaged soul to reach the afterlife. But as the concept of the sanctity of life strengthened, suicide became more of an abomination, and the penalties decreed by the church became more severe. It became a cardinal sin: the suicide was refused Christian burial, the body was desecrated, and the family publicly humiliated. If the suicide left a fortune, the church seized it and rendered the family destitute.

The doctrine of the church prohibiting suicide remained unchallenged until the Renaissance. In 1516, Sir Thomas More, in *Utopia,* raised the issue of voluntary euthanasia, or suicide, for people who had incurable and painful diseases. A century later, Francis Bacon suggested that it was a physician's duty to help a patient "make a faire and easy passage." The following centuries brought increasingly probing discussion of euthanasia, both pro and con, by numerous philosophers and writers.[20] John Donne, Montaigne, Voltaire, Rousseau, Montesquieu, Hume, and Bentham all wrote in favor of suicide, while Kant, Schopenhauer, Nietzsche, and William James opposed it.

It is tempting to see disagreement over suicide and physician-assisted dying as a clash between religious and secular views. But in fact there is a variety of purely religious views on the same subject.[21] With its tradition as a sanctuary for the religiously persecuted, the United States now harbors a wide range of structured religions; some accept rational suicide, others openly oppose it, and still others are publicly neutral on the subject.[22]

The Unitarian Universalist Church has been outspokenly in favor of rational suicide and physician-assisted dying for certain medical conditions and has given strong support to state referenda in Washington, California, and Oregon. This church has strong feelings about the dignity of human life and the absolute and inviolable right to self-determination. Its resolution in 1988 stated that "Unitarian Universalists advocate the right to self-determination in dying and the release from civil and criminal penalties for those who, under proper safeguards, act to honor the right for terminally ill patients to select the time of their own deaths."[23]

Opposition to any form of suicide and physician-assisted dying comes from fundamentalist groups, the religious right, and other conservative religious groups. Roman Catholicism, Christian Science, Jehovah's Witnesses, Judaism, the Eastern Orthodox churches, the United Pentecostal Church, the Mormon Church, the Church of the Nazarene, and the Episcopal, Lutheran, and Southern Baptist churches all have doctrinal proscriptions against suicide. Islam also opposes suicide for any reason.

This leaves a large number of churches and religious groups that have maintained a neutral silence on the issue. Foremost among these are the United Church of Christ and the Presbyterian Church, both of which place strong emphasis on individual freedom and responsibility and the right to choose. Members of the Presbyterian clergy have spoken out in favor of physician-assisted dying, but the council has preferred not to make a statement.[24] Other churches that take no absolute stand on the issue include the Adventists, most Baptist churches, the Christian Reformed Church of North America, the Church of Christ, and the Pentecostal Church of God. Some of these have no central authoritative body to speak on such matters, leaving these responsibilities to the individual congregations. Others have consciously decided to avoid the subject until the legal aspects of it have been better defined. They do not feel justified in trying to influence social policy, and their silence perhaps represents watchful waiting rather than moral conviction in either direction.

The Jewish View Based on the Hebrew Scriptures, Jewish teaching has historically opposed abortion and suicide, and hence assisted dying.[25] According to this creed, every moment of human life has infinite value. Not only is life a gift from God, but so is the body that it inhabits. Nothing can compromise this principle, which is more important in Orthodox Jewish thinking than personal autonomy. Suffering must be accepted, and the physician's role is to provide healing. No exception is made for a body that lives devoid of useful function and productivity. The possible exception is the person who is terminally ill—that is, in the process of dying. Controversy has arisen over the definition of *terminal* and the issue of "brain death," when respiration is supported artificially but the heart is still beating. Withdrawing technical support (the respirator) is debatable, but discontinuing nourishment and hydration is not allowed.

The strict views of Orthodox Jews are softened somewhat in the thinking of Conservative Judaism, where removal of life-sustaining nutrition is now the focus of discussion. Reformed Judaism places much greater emphasis on autonomy, considering abortion, for example, to be a personal decision. Quality of life is an important consideration and the role of the physician is broader but does not include any action that deliberately shortens life.

The Roman Catholic View By far the most influential voice against suicide in the Western world is that of the Roman Catholic Church.[26] The Catholic proscription against any suicide, including assisted suicide, was first stated by St. Augustine. Man, he wrote, was created in the image of God and blessed with a special relationship because of the perfection of this image. Through respect for this image and this relationship, one gained immortality and the joys of afterlife. Martyrdom was virtuous only when it was done out of devotion to God and not for selfish reasons. Augustine found particular infamy in the killing of an innocent person: "For it is clear that if no one has a private right to kill even a guilty man (and no law allows this), then certainly anyone who kills himself is a murderer, and is the more guilty in killing himself the more innocent he is of the charge on which he has condemned himself to death."[27]

St. Thomas Aquinas expanded on this with views that are repeated today almost verbatim by the modern Roman Catholic Church:

1. Everything in nature loves and protects itself. Suicide is contrary to natural law.
2. Every man is part of the community, so in killing himself he injures the community.
3. Life is God's gift to man. Whoever takes his own life sins against God.

4. The passage from this life to another and happier one is subject not to man's free will but to the power of God.[28]

Today's Religious Debate The current basis for religious opposition to suicide and physician-assisted dying still follows two major lines. The first of these is the sanctity of life: all life, but particularly human life, is recognized as a direct gift from God, but a special gift, one that never becomes personal property. It is ours not to give away, to damage, or to destroy at will, but to preserve intact until the moment when it is taken back. These arguments can seem persuasive and acceptable when the life is a happy and healthy one, but such beliefs can be severely stressed in the presence of advanced and painful disease. At that point the gift may no longer be wanted and the loan gladly repaid. The notion of a divinely prescribed duration of the loan is also challenged by the success of modern medicine in markedly prolonging life. A strict interpretation of the limits of life would negate all that is expected of physicians.

The second and peculiarly Christian belief regarding death is that suffering can be beneficial in its own right. Suffering that cannot be avoided should be cast in a positive light, thus perhaps making it more bearable. St. Paul said that "we welcome our sufferings." The Lutheran Church has declared that "God can work the gift of grace for the one who suffers and for others."[29] Similarly, the Vatican declaration on euthanasia states that "suffering during the last moments of life is in fact a sharing in Christ's passion." In fact, "It is rather the mark of a good and Holy God that He permits so many of His children to undergo that suffering here on Earth. Suffering is almost the greatest gift of God's love."[30] An extension of this thinking is that suffering is a result of guilt that leads to repentance. The greater the suffering, the greater the guilt, hence the greater the need for repentance. Conversely, any attempt to avoid suffering lessens the opportunity to repent. An associate of mine described a young woman who was dying of ovarian cancer but insisted on more and more aggressive treatment long after there was any hope for cure or even prolonged survival. She continued to push her physicians to do more, even when her situation was clearly hopeless. She finally confided to a nurse that she was terrified of dying because her past sins had been so great that she was sure that any afterlife would be most unpleasant.

This argument has been extended to the concept of courage and fortitude in language that I would find difficult to present to a patient: "Precisely because they want to escape suffering, immature people attempt to control reality and refuse to be shaped by its demands. . . . Suffering can bring self-transcendence by breaking down the rigid and introverted ego. . . . Seeking to control and to master death by making it our servant, forcing it to serve at our convenience, and subordinating it to our egotistical concerns is a failure to be open to reality and a failure to be mature spiritually. Accepting death and suffering on its own terms is a sign of full psychological integrity, spiritual maturity, and confidence in Christ."[31]

These arguments, of course, fall on deaf ears for those who do not embrace the underlying faith. They are also challenged by those who do share the faith when the suffering seems out of proportion to any possible spiritual benefit. The reality of serious and painful illness can cause even the most devout Christian to question God's goodness, to ask, "What have I done to deserve so much pain?" Only an unfeeling observer can equate cowardice and uncertainty in the face of painful disease. Indeed, many contemplate suicide but pull back from the act for lack of courage to go through with it. As we shall see, some ethicists favor physician-assisted suicide over euthanasia precisely because it places greater responsibility—with a corresponding requirement for courage—on the shoulders of the patient. Finally, there is the obvious medical truism that suffering, if considered an intrinsic good, is amply available throughout life. Indeed, the church opposed the use of analgesia for childbirth when it was first introduced on the grounds that God intended delivery to be painful. Now analgesia for childbirth and for many other conditions is expected rather than just accepted.

As we have seen, Helga Kuhse has challenged "sanctity of life" as an absolute doctrine both because it is inconsistent and because it fails to consider quality of life. In her view, "What is important is not that a patient is human (and therefore should have her life sustained). Rather we must ask questions about the quality and kind of the patient's life. . . . Life may be in a being's interests, or it may not—depending on what the life is like. . . . The question is not whether decisions to end human lives should sometimes be made; rather the question is on what principle or principles these inevitable life and death decisions should be made."[32]

Margaret Battin, professor of philosophy at the University of Utah, has noted that some religious beliefs based on the concept of an afterlife can be construed as invitations to suicide: "Eternal reunion with parents, close relatives, and even friends, may have special appeal to those who are slowly dying because of the associated promise of loving care and comfort." She observes that "the early release of the immortal soul from a crumbling, tortured body could be a very desirable separation."[33]

W. R. Matthews, dean of St. Paul's Cathedral in London from 1934 to 1967, wrote, "The great master principle of love and its offshoot, compassion, would permit an adult person of sound mind whose life is ending with much suffering, to choose between an easy death and a hard one, and to obtain medical aid in implementing that choice."[34]

Finally, even within religious groups that are strongly opposed to any form of suicide and physician-assisted dying, there are exceptions. Daniel Maguire, a Catholic philosopher in the department of theology at Marquette University, has written, "In a medical context, it may be moral and should be legal to accelerate the death process by taking direct action."[35] He quotes Aquinas's dictum that "human actions are good or bad according to their circumstances," then criticizes current Catholic teaching for its "strong temptation to ignore this rudimentary insight into the morally differentiating meaning of circumstances." In cases where we sense moral uncertainty, the religious community frequently retreats to the simplistics of taboo. "The taboo mentality considers certain classes of actions bad 'regardless of the circumstances.' The stimulus for taboo comes from the perceived security of knowing that what cannot be used, cannot be abused." But "taboo knows no exceptions, and that is its weakness."

The Catholic Church is experiencing a widening gap between its official and often archaic doctrine and the thinking and practices of today's membership, with the clergy sometimes acting as a buffer between the two. A hospital chaplain whom I interviewed explained his liberal position that his ministerial responsibility is to support individuals in their own decisions, even if they differ from the teachings if the Church. "The people who tell us what we should do are far from the grim reality of the hospital bedside. I am in the trenches, dealing every day with people who are suffering and dying, and asking for understanding and forgiveness and for merciful deaths. And that's what they should get." Catholic priests have even been known to take pleas for mercy into their own hands. In seventeenth-century Brittany, seriously ill patients could ask for the "holy stone," with which a priest administered a crushing blow to the head of the suffering victim.[36]

Catholics in the latter half of the twentieth century have contended with the issues of divorce and birth control and are now struggling with abortion. Public opinion polls show that Catholics are almost as likely to favor physician-assisted dying as is the general population. Beyond that, the rapid spread of information and conflicting views in a secular and questioning society is drawing many Catholics away from previously held religious beliefs and rigid dogma. Arguments built around the sanctity of life and religious aspects of suffering have their adherents but have limited appeal to the general public. Religious suffering is not for everyone. The result is that conservative religious groups are now framing their objections in more secular language and concepts, invoking the possibility of abuse and the theoretical slippery slope toward social decay. Courtney Campbell cites a problem in translation inherent in this new strategy: "Once translated for purposes of public debate, the religious influence seems, at best, indirect and perhaps dispensable."[37] The sponsorship of these religious objections is harder to disguise. The Catholic Church contributed large amounts of money to try to defeat the ballot measures that were voted on in Washington, California, and Oregon.

THE LAW

Religious influence over political bodies was strong in the Middle Ages, and the prohibition against suicide was enacted into law as a crime against the state as well as the church. As states became more powerful, they seized from the church the right to the property of the suicide and his family. These conditions persisted for a remarkably long time. Well into the nineteenth century in England, the body of a suicide was placed at the intersection of a crossroads with a stake driven through the corpse for all to see.[38]

The position of the state and its bond to the church was encapsulated by Blackstone: "The suicide is guilty of a double offense. One spiritual, invading the prerogative of the Almighty and rushing into His immediate presence uncalled for; the other, temporal, against the king, who hath an interest in the preservation of all his subjects."[39] The legal echo of this was provided by the Missouri Supreme Court in its ruling on Nancy Cruzan: "The state's interest is not in quality of life. . . . Instead, the state's interest is in life; that interest is unqualified."[40]

It should be noted that the original decriminalization of suicide in the 1960s in no way reflected approval of suicide by the lawmakers. Two key reasons for this reversal were the impossibility of prosecuting a person who is dead and the patent unfairness of depriving the innocent family of the suicide's possessions. More important, if a suicidal person is considered incompetent, by definition he cannot have committed a criminal act. Finally, the medical rehabilitation of the attempted suicide is more logical and promising if the act has no criminal onus attached to it. The Catholic Church has also recognized the medical aspects of suicide and now grants these people Christian burial. Similarly, most insurance companies consider suicide to be an acceptable cause of death once a certain term has passed—typically two years—since the policy was purchased.

The courts have gone to great lengths to avoid ruling on the legality of suicide, even when patients have elected to terminate medical care or support. In most cases the patient's choice was interpreted as the rejection of unwanted apparatus and encumbrances, even though death was the obvious consequence. The law is still very uneasy with the entire concept of suicide and is only beginning to grapple with the basic issue of rational suicide.

The Medicalization of Suicide

The advent of Christianity didn't bring an end to rational suicide, of course, though to some extent the practice was forced "into the closet." Several public figures in the twentieth century are thought to have died with medical assistance. King George V of England was helped to die by his personal physician, Lord Dawson of Penn, through the use of a fatal dose of morphine and cocaine. Lord Dawson was granted permission by the royal family to "act at any moment to end a painful death." Sigmund Freud suffered from cancer of the throat and eventually prevailed upon his physician to give him a lethal dose of narcotics.[41] And more recently, though only close family members know the truth, the circumstances surrounding the death of Jacqueline Kennedy Onassis suggest that hers was a planned death, with or without the help of a physician. To me, her illness, non-Hodgkins lymphoma, did not seem to be advanced enough to be terminal. She was photographed walking in Central Park shortly before she died. Moreover, her entire family was present at the time of her death, and the next day her son announced that she did it "in her own way." It is fair to speculate that she ended her dignified life with an equally dignified death.

Still, in spite of these manifestly sane decisions to end life, the concept has evolved throughout the nineteenth century and into the twentieth that suicide is a manifestation of mental disturbance and that the individual is not responsible for his or her action. This resulted in decriminalization of suicide in England in 1965 and in all of the United States by the mid-1970s. This principle grew out of the observation that many suicides occurred in patients who had severe manic depressive (biphasic) disorders, those who were under severe emotional stress, and those who had suffered psychological trauma. By many estimates, 90 percent of all suicides or suicide attempts are secondary to mental illness. The common denominator in most of these situations is depression. Psychiatric interest in suicide was reinforced by the success of treating depression with psychotherapy and electroconvulsive therapy, and the even greater success of new antidepressant drugs. Indeed, depression is now one of the illnesses most successfully treated by psychologists and psychiatrists, with success rates higher than 80 percent.

Suicide is a major public health problem, with more than thirty thousand reported in the United States each year and a significant number going unreported.[42] It is the eighth leading cause of death for all ages, and fourth in young adults, exceeded in males only by accidents, homicide, and AIDS. The highest rate, however, is among white males in their eighties; complicating risk factors include living alone, alcoholism, social isolation, and previous suicide attempts.

Medicalization of suicide has led to the mistaken concept that suicidal thoughts are always symptoms of depression and that depression can always be treated. No normal person, the argument goes, would try to kill himself: "When a terminally ill patient contemplates suicide, it usually means he or she is suffering from an irrational thought process, characteristic of a major clinical depression, not solely from the terminal illness."[43]

The average psychiatrist has little experience with people who have serious physical illness, and very few have experience with dying patients in hospice or cancer hospital settings, where dispassionate discussion of rational suicide is apt to take place. Psychiatrists are much more frequently called upon to evaluate and treat purely or predominantly psychiatric disorders. A psychiatrist who works primarily in the emergency setting explained that "the manual for the diagnosis of depression really does not concern itself with the etiology. Whether it's primary or secondary to life circumstances, when we're diagnosing depression we're looking for symptoms and signs, and then, if the diagnosis is met, a treatment. The factors which contribute to depression are important, but for the actual treatment, the etiology may not have any bearing."

Depression associated with terminal illness may be completely impervious to treatment in the face of the advancing disease. Moreover, psychotherapy is a slow process, and antidepressant drugs take several weeks to be effective, by which time the patient may have succumbed to the disease.[44] Patients who have no past experience with personality disorders or depression may be insulted even by the suggestion of psychiatric treatment and may refuse any offered therapy.

Psychiatrists and psychologists are also in a difficult position. The reluctance of many even to consider rational suicide may drive away potential patients whose depression could and should be treated. The notion of complicity in rational suicide gives even an experienced psychiatrist pause. If asked to see a seriously ill patient who is talking about taking his own life, the psychiatrist might feel obliged to intervene, if only because of the potential legal problems should the patient kill himself after the consultation. One of my associates explained his duties as follows:

> My responsibilities are to diagnose and to treat and to prevent this man from causing himself harm, despite the fact that I might feel he does not have a mood disorder or anxiety disorder. If I thought he was going to walk out of this office and kill himself I would probably have the police bring him over to the hospital. I would have him wait in the waiting room and

call his wife to get the gun or the pills. I would try to protect him from those impulses. We walk a terrible, litigious line right now. I would be forced to infringe seriously on his civil rights, but that is the thorny dilemma and dichotomy that we find ourselves in. It is standard practice to view this as a pathological process and try to intervene in it.[45]

Central to our consideration of rational suicide and assisted dying is the relation between serious physical illness and suicide. Chronic or terminal illnesses are often statistically linked to suicide; physical illness is considered to be a significant factor in as many as 25 percent of all cases. Cancer and AIDS are the "bad deaths" most frequently associated with suicidal impulses. It is not clear how common or uncommon spoken suicidal thoughts are in cancer patients. Emanuel reported that 27 percent of 155 oncology patients questioned had entertained serious thoughts about requesting assisted suicide or euthanasia and that 12 percent had initiated such discussion with their physicians or families.[46] On the other hand, Brown and associates conducted a study in which only 3 of 44 patients with late-stage cancer were found to have considered suicide, and each of them was thought to be suffering from severe clinical depression.[47] I don't think that this latter study gives a clear picture of the concern that seriously ill patients have about how their lives might end. Many more may consider suicide in private, without ever making their feelings known.

I interviewed several cancer patients in preparing to write this book. Most were in favor of laws that would permit physicians to help them die and said that they might take advantage of such help, were it available. A few of the patients were terminally ill. All expressed sadness that life would end so soon. One had received treatment in the past for clinical depression and alcoholism. At the time of my interview, however, she was not depressed; on the contrary, she was outgoing and pleased about placing her terminal care in the hands of a friend at the Connecticut Hospice. Another had a history of severe depressive reactions whenever she received bad news about her illness, reactions that ended as soon as she began to feel better. The remaining patients had no histories of clinical depression, nor did they show any signs of depression that I could detect during my interviews or that their treating physicians were aware of. All denied having had or having wanted any treatment for depression. At least one of the patients did eventually take her own life, by self-imposed starvation.

What, then, is the difference between the patients in Brown's study, whose thoughts of suicide were rare and confined to people with severe clinical depression, and the people whom I interviewed, who were not apparently depressed but who spoke openly of thoughts of taking their own lives and of the desirability of having help available? One possibility is that the people whom I interviewed were self-selected for willingness to discuss assisted dying with me. They were thought by all to be emotionally intact at the time, and none was under observation or treatment for depression or suicidal tendencies. Another difference may have been the exact topic being discussed. For many people, suicide conveys a repulsive picture of violence, while assisted dying is much more gentle in concept and in fact. Indeed, some opponents of assisted dying feel that introducing compassionate medical help would make the act too easy for the patient. The ability to have not only a peaceful death but a clean, nonviolent one would remove a strong psychological barrier. Patients who are dying may stop short of taking their own lives because of the additional trauma to themselves and their families. Already sick and perhaps dirty in their own eyes, they have little desire to make things worse through violence. Fatigue from fighting disease may also leave insufficient energy to pursue an end to life without outside help. Indeed, the need for help may explain why relatively few people who are dying of fatal illnesses attempt to end their lives. They wait so long that they cannot do it alone. Finally, many people may be reluctant to discuss suicidal thoughts with mental health professionals because of a purely rational recognition that expressing their thoughts in our current medical, legal, and moral climate is futile. Discussing the possibility of suicide with family or physician may mean that any plan will be immediately thwarted.

In a moving article describing his mother's experience with cancer and eventual suicide, Andrew Solomon said that "having been through the whole business, I would put the infrequency of suicide down more to the difficulty of it than to the undesirability of its objectives."[48] The discrepancies among various reports underline the need for much larger and more probing studies of the degree to which serious physical illness can inspire considerations of rational suicide or physician-assisted dying, particularly in the absence of any previous documented mental illness.

Public acceptance of rational suicide requires recognizing that not all contemplations of suicide are the same. It is essential to consider the main reasons for wishing to die to see the difference. The underlying issues remain the autonomous right of the individual to avoid unnecessary suffering.

A doctor brought me into this world, and others have certainly helped me throughout my life, particularly with this illness. It seems perfectly reasonable that a doctor should help me end my life when the time comes. *A cancer patient*

3 The Search for Help: Physician Assistance

Although individuals and families dealing with end-of-life issues frequently need help, this help often has not been forthcoming from the expected source—namely, the medical profession. Today's medicine is still much more oriented toward aggressive treatment than it is toward moderating distress at the end of life. This has led to the development of three quite different sources of help for the dying: directives, comfort care, and assisted dying.

Directives

The several forms of directives include written advance directives, by which a person determines what restrictions, if any, he would like to place on his medical care if he becomes incompetent; the designation of a surrogate with durable power of attorney to make decisions for him or to enforce the written directive; and "do not resuscitate" (DNR) orders that the patient or a family member or surrogate makes near the end of the patient's life. All three options are designed primarily to limit the amount of medical intervention that can be used to prolong life.[1] DNR orders, the simplest of the three options, forbid the use of cardiac and/or pulmonary resuscitation at a time of impending death. These orders are based on the understanding that the person has an underlying fatal disease and that death is expected; the orders can be requested by a competent patient, his appointed surrogate, or members of his family. Advance directives, or living wills, are usually prepared in times of relatively good health and full mental competence to cover future circumstances when serious illness may compromise that competence. One's autonomy can be further extended through a durable power of attorney. This is usually vested in a close relative or friend who can be trusted to speak for the patient.

There are two problems with all of these forms of directives: many people do not take the time to prepare them, and many physicians do not pay any attention to them. The physician may be unaware of her patient's preferences, or she may simply succumb to the reflexive dismissal of such attention to patient autonomy as contrary to the traditional role and responsibility of medicine.[2] The physician may also fear legal liability if she does the wrong thing. Needless to say, if physicians tend to ignore DNR orders in the face of impending death, they are going to be even less responsive to advance directives or surrogates designated in the remote past, under entirely different circumstances.

A revealing and disturbing study was carried out in five medical centers on what should be the simplest of these directives, DNR orders.[3] The first phase of the study confirmed that there were substantial shortcomings in the care of seriously ill patients in intensive care units: some physicians did not know whether their patients wished to avoid resuscitation, some were very slow to write DNR orders, and some kept dying patients in intensive care for a prolonged time. In addition, family members reported that patients suffered severe pain for several days at a time. More disturbing, though, was the second phase of this study, in which a concerted effort was made to counteract these deficiencies, with little improvement. The study concluded that "Enhancing opportunities for more patient-physician communication, although advocated as the major method for improving patient outcomes, may be inadequate to change established practices. To improve the experience of seriously ill and dying patients, greater individual and societal commitment and more proactive and forceful measures may be needed." Indeed, medical education must place far greater emphasis on the needs of the dying patient.

Comfort Care

Most chronic or fatal illnesses eventually reach a point where further active treatment is futile and burdensome, and the goals of curing the disease and prolonging life are best abandoned in favor of providing comfort. Under the stimulus of the hospice program, methods for providing comfort have been developed and the value of such care is becoming increasingly well recognized. The purpose of comfort care is to relieve pain and all other symptoms, including anxiety, to the extent that medication and personal support make it possible. For the same reason that expensive and aggressive treatment is being abandoned, acute care hospitals are usually not the best places to attempt to provide comfort care. This type of care is better given in less pressured environments: homes, nursing homes, or residential hospice institutions. Implicit in comfort care is the understanding that it will be given continuously to the very end, that the patient will not be abandoned by his caregivers. Physicians have much to learn about comfort care, and some have begun to educate themselves, possibly under the "threat" of legalized assisted dying.

The model for comfort care is the hospice program.[4] Originating in medieval times, a hospice was traditionally a stopping place for pilgrims and travelers, where they could receive shelter and refreshment. Those who were ill, injured, or exhausted could stay until they were able to resume their journeys. The Irish Sisters of Charity opened Our Lady's Hospice in Dublin in 1846 and St. Joseph's Hospice in London in 1905. Both became so identified with the care of the dying that the term *hospice* acquired a new meaning. The modern day hospice program was started in 1967 by Cicely Saunders at St. Christopher's Hospice in London as an alternative to being hospitalized at the end of life. The first residential hospice in the United States was opened in 1974 in Branford, Connecticut, by Dr. Sylvia Lack. The hospice movement developed rapidly, and the United States now has about 2,500 home hospice programs, in which care is provided by visiting nurses with special hospice training, and 200 residential hospice facilities.

The philosophy of hospice is to keep dying patients as comfortable as possible through the control of pain and other symptoms, but neither to prolong life nor to hasten death. Although the care obviously centers around the patient, the entire family is involved. Supportive measures are limited to those that contribute directly to providing comfort, and all others are excluded. Most laboratory studies are eliminated, and drawing of blood is avoided if at all possible. X-rays are not taken unless they will influence the care being given. Nutrition and hydration are usually limited to what can be taken by mouth. Tube feedings and intravenous feeding are not started, but may be continued if they are already in place. Blood transfusions are not given, and oxygen is only provided when it is needed to provide comfort. Mechanical ventilation is not used.

The high level of care given by hospice programs is provided primarily through expert nursing, with careful attention to the control of pain and other symptoms, hygiene, care for wounds and the mouth, and so on. Behind the dedicated nursing care in residential hospice facilities is an interdisciplinary support team that includes a physician and a social worker, and that makes available counseling and religious support for patients and families. In home hospice care programs the visiting hospice nurse is usually the only direct con-

nection to the program. The patient's primary physician, who is outside of the hospice program, remains in charge. The nurse may refer problems to the hospice physician, but the hospice physician
rarely if ever sees the patient at home.

The hospice program received a tremendous boost when it
was brought under the financial umbrella of Medicare and Medicaid. In addition to providing a stable source of money for most patients, this accreditation also establishes standards of care and rules
to control costs. Among the cost-control measures is the requirement that 80 percent of the care be given at home, with a residential
hospice used only at the end of the illness, if at all. Life expectancy
for the person admitted to the hospice program, at home or in a residential unit, is set at six months or less. This must be agreed upon
by the referring physician and the hospice physician. On entering
the hospice program under the auspices of Medicare, the patient
and family must accept the philosophy of hospice to provide comfort care only, acknowledging the fatal nature of the disease. Originally, hospice care was provided primarily for cancer patients. In recent years it has been extended to AIDS and many other chronic but
fatal diseases, but even now about 80 percent of hospice patients
have cancer.

Our knowledge and appreciation of comfort care has expanded
enormously under the stimulation of hospice programs. The movement is now well established, and it is certain to continue to grow
and be a major provider of end-of-life care. Still, the hospice program has its own limitations. The first of these is the inherent dis-
continuity of care at the end of life. The patient with cancer, for example, may be followed for years by an appropriate specialist or
family practitioner. When active treatment is given up or rejected, a
home care program is usually instituted. The home hospice program
provides a gradual transition from active treatment to comfort care.
This phase of the illness is managed by the original physician, who
continues to do so until the patient becomes too ill to travel to the
office or clinic. At this point, direct contact with his regular physi-

cian usually ends, though the hospice nurse may refer to the physician regularly. If death takes place at home, it is overseen by the visiting nurse, unless a family physician is involved. The absence of the original physician can seem like abandonment to some patients and family members.

Transfer of a person to a residential hospice entails an abrupt and complete change of circumstances. All previous physicians and health care personnel are replaced, and the last days or weeks of life are passed in new surroundings with new people. It is not surprising that many people may see this as further abandonment, not only by their physicians and nurses but also by their families, who can no longer take care of them at home. Because the transfer is put off as long as possible, the patient sometimes arrives at hospice essentially moribund, with only a few days or even hours to live.

The Connecticut Hospice facility is attractive, and the care and understanding that hospice can provide for the dying far exceeds that of most acute care hospitals. For some patients and families, dying at home is physically or emotionally impossible to deal with, and hospice fills an important void. But acknowledging that hospice is "where you go to die" can be very upsetting. The patient may have not only his own death to contend with but the deaths of others, perhaps even in the next bed. The hospice patient is surrounded by death. Patients and families alike who anticipate the possibility of using a hospice institution should try to visit it first, to ease the future transition and to be sure that it is a step that they really wish to take. Dying at home, in familiar surroundings with family members at hand, may be a better alternative for some.

Although hospice does very well in providing control of pain and symptoms for most people, the best of care occasionally fails.[5] Several hospice caregivers whom I have spoken to have acknowledged that in spite of all efforts, some of their patients suffer severely at the end of life. Hospice caregivers know that they cannot guarantee a pain-free, dignified death. They see at first hand suffering that is difficult to control and acknowledge that stupefying doses of narcotics are occasionally used to kill pain at the expense of dignity and autonomy and with the understanding that death may be brought on sooner. Indeed, requests for earlier death are not uncommon. The standard reply is "We can't." Even though patients may ask for assistance in dying, hospice policies forbid it, and their patients have no alternative but to "live until they die." Hospice has embraced the concept of patient autonomy, but not to the point of allowing assisted dying.

The current discussion of physician-assisted dying has seriously challenged the hospice principle of not shortening life, and hospice leaders have officially taken a very defensive position against any consideration of this activity. One reason for this stance is that many hospice programs are closely allied to and supported by the Catholic Church. Another reason is related to ambivalence about the so-called double effect. According to that principle, it is permissible to prescribe drugs for an acceptable purpose in the knowledge that they may have secondary effects that are technically unacceptable. Much of the public and many physicians believe that the use by hospices of heavy doses of narcotics to relieve pain under the principle of the double effect comes perilously close to assisted dying. Because earlier death is often the result, the acceptability of this practice hinges on intent. Public acceptance of intentionally helping people die would make it very hard for the hospice system to maintain its practice and philosophy. Finally, there is a perceived financial conflict of interest. People who elect assisted dying at home will obviously not be candidates for residential hospice, and some fear that assisted dying will totally eclipse the hospice movement. This seems unlikely to me. Hospice already cares for and benefits many people very well. The number who would seek an alternative should not be expected to be large enough to undermine the hospice system. Moreover, hospices are much too well established to be destroyed by legalization of assisted dying. Instead, I think the hospice system will find a way to broaden its own philosophy.

Even now there may be a drift away from the original hard line of hospice thinking. I have met hospice workers, and even directors, who have participated in meetings to promote assisted dying, acknowledging their personal views that hospices should someday embrace this concept. One study of hospice physicians and ethics panel members showed that only half would oppose assisted suicide if it were legal, and even fewer if active euthanasia were permissible. Only 45 percent would oppose efforts to decriminalize either of these steps.[6]

The development of comfort care and hospice to extend medical help to the terminally ill and their families is one of the great health care advances in several Western countries, particularly Great Britain and the United States. As a profession, physicians must increase their level of personal responsibility for their patients, right up to the point of death. Caring and compassion cannot be turned off when treatment fails, because treatment always eventually fails in terminal illness. The hospice movement is held up as an alternative to assisted dying, and so it should be. But to speak of an alternative is to imply that there is a choice, and at the present time the leaders of the hospice movement are determined to see that there is no alternative and therefore no choice. Discussion with patients, home hospice nurses, and hospice physicians indicates that a significant number of patients would prefer to die at home and that some among them would like to have physician assistance in bringing their lives to an end. Hospice is not for everyone. Moreover, the increasing and welcome emphasis on palliation does not mean that a person is required to pursue this approach until it is exhausted. He has every right to refuse any form of treatment or care, including prolonged palliative care.

Private and Public Acceptance

Public concern about how life may end has brought progressive developments on three fronts: organizations have emerged to provide information on assisted dying, some physicians have acknowledged that they have been approached and have provided help to patients who wanted to die, and public opinion polls have revealed growing acceptance for more liberal laws governing the end of life.

ORGANIZATIONS

Although it was not the first organization to promote euthanasia and assisted suicide, the Hemlock Society was the first such major effort in the United States.[7] Founded in 1980 by Derrick Humphrey, the society originally had two missions: to provide specific information to interested individuals, and to promote appropriate legislation. As a source of information, the society's efforts reached their peak with the publication of Humphrey's *Final Exit,* a "how-to" book on suicide that became a best-seller.[8] The impressive sales for this book gave some indication of the interest among the general public in having control over their final days. Following that publication, the Hemlock Society retreated somewhat from providing direct information in order to concentrate on public education and to lobby for more liberal legislation. The society gave particular attention to the three western states that had referenda on assisted dying—California, Washington, and Oregon—and to other states where changes in legislation were being considered. Through its many state and local chapters and numerous publications, the Hemlock Society has assumed the leading role in public education about assisted dying.

A splinter group from the Hemlock Society, Compassion in Dying, expanded on Hemlock's original missions, both at the bedside and in the courts.[9] This society was founded in 1993, in the wake of the defeat of Washington's assisted-death proposition. The society was founded by Rev. Ralph Mero, a Unitarian Universalist minister, who also was one of the founders of the Washington State division of Hemlock. In addition to providing information on assisted death to appropriate patients, Compassion in Dying helps patients find doctors who may be willing to write the required prescriptions, but the organization does not provide the materials. More important, the group offers to have a volunteer present, not to help with the dying but to support patient and family at the time of death.[10] Compassion in Dying limits its activities to patients who are terminally ill and who are able to obtain appropriate drugs from their own doctors. It encourages patients and physicians to collaborate in finding a way to an earlier and more comfortable death.

Compassion in Dying took an enormous legal step in challenging the constitutionality of the Washington law forbidding physicians from assisting patients to die. The challenge was eventually upheld in the Ninth Circuit Court of Appeals, which agreed that the existing laws were unconstitutional. A similar case, also sponsored by Compassion in Dying, was brought up in New York State, with the same result. These two cases were later appealed by their respective states to the U.S. Supreme Court, which reversed the opinions of the lower courts and upheld the existing laws.

PHYSICIANS

Jack Kevorkian is a retired pathologist. His professional life never included any responsibility for people who had fatal diseases, but his name is now associated with physician-assisted dying in the minds of most of the American public. In June 1990, Kevorkian assisted in the suicide of his first patient, Janet Adkins, who had Alzheimer's disease. Since then he has assisted in more than one hundred deaths for a wide range of problems. Some patients, like Mrs. Adkins, were clearly not terminal, nor were they suffering severe pain. His assistance has always required activation of some device by the patient, presumably to avoid the more serious legal problems of euthanasia.

Kevorkian's activities have troubled physicians and ethicists, even some who favor assisted dying. Critics decry his seeming quest for publicity, his idiosyncratic process and criteria for patient selection, his lack of clinical knowledge of the patients' earlier diseases, and his relatively short-term association with his patients. But he is highly regarded by many patients, their families, and even the general public. A patient of mine berated her husband because he could not find "a Dr. Kevorkian" to help her end her life when she was dying of pancreatic cancer. Three acquittals on murder charges have made it clear that jurors in Michigan felt that his activities were justified. Indeed, his prosecutor in Wayne County, John D. O'Hare, also proposed a bill that would legalize doctor-assisted suicide in that state, stating that if he himself were terminally ill, he would "not have a moment's hesitation" in seeking a doctor's help in ending his own life.

Timothy Quill brought a new perspective to physician-assisted dying, one that was much less abrasive to the sensitivities of the medical profession. His background as an oncologist and hospice physician provided him with firsthand experience with patients who had terminal illnesses. In a landmark article in the *New England Journal of Medicine,* Quill described his assistance in the death of Diane, a long-term patient of his who had leukemia.[11] She feared increasing discomfort and dependence on others, and had a strong desire to control the time and place of her own death. She had an experienced and sympathetic physician in Quill. After long discussions he gave her prescriptions for barbiturates "for sleep," realizing that she would probably use them to take her own life. He was convinced that she was rational and not depressed and wished primarily to secure death on her own terms. Two days after their final meeting, she did just that, on the couch in her own house, after saying good-bye to her husband and son and asking them to leave her alone. Quill poignantly wondered "why Diane, who gave so much to so many of us, had to be alone for the last hour of her life."

Timothy Quill's rich clinical experience and high standing in the medical community place him in an entirely different category from Jack Kevorkian. He has gone on to write two books on the subject of assisted dying and has participated as one of the plaintiffs in the case that went to the Second Circuit Court of Appeals and then on to the U.S. Supreme Court.[12]

Finally, the general public has increasingly expressed its support for laws that would permit physician-assisted dying. Several studies have shown that about 65 percent of respondents favor laws that would permit some form of assisted dying, up from 36 percent in 1950. A summary of several large polls published in 1992 showed that 63 percent of those contacted favored physician-assisted dying.[13] Surprisingly, this view was shared by about the same proportion of the Catholic and Protestant populations. A much smaller number, 24 percent, thought that they would personally ask their physicians to help them end their own lives if their distress was great enough. A study of the surviving close relatives of 1,144 people who died in Utah in 1992 showed that 17 percent thought that the deceased would have elected assisted dying if it had been legally available.[14] A poll of more than 8,000 Americans showed that highly educated, politically liberal people whose religious beliefs were not strong were the most likely to favor some form of assisted dying. Moreover, the majority preferred the idea of active euthanasia over physician-assisted suicide.[15]

Physician Assistance

Medical treatment carries the promise of curing disease, a promise that is often fulfilled. If the disease cannot be cured, life may be prolonged at a reasonable level of comfort. Eventually that may fail, and the patient turns again to the physician for help. An unfortunate few encounter suffering that is beyond their endurance. More than ever, they need help—help, now, not to live but to die. The most appropriate people to provide assistance in dying have always been physicians. Over the centuries they have quietly provided help out of sympathy and compassion. Physician-assisted deaths have usually taken place at home, in complete privacy, when patient, family, and physician agreed that there was nothing to be gained by allowing the dying process to linger. Recently the absolute bans on suicide, both religious and legal, have been relaxed, and we are seeing renewed concern about the role of physician assistance.[16]

The physician is also the obvious choice because she has access to the necessary drugs, most of which can be obtained only by prescription. Furthermore, the physician who lacks the necessary information can obtain it. Many patients interviewed for this study saw physician-assisted dying as a needed extension of relief from suffering and as a form of caring. If sympathy and support at the time of dying are acts of compassion, then actual help is surely even more so.

It has been suggested that responsibility for assistance in dying should be given to people outside of the medical profession, even to the point of developing a new profession of people who specialize in helping others die. The implication is that assisted dying may be acceptable in principle but that it is not an appropriate role for physicians. Some who suggest transferring the responsibility outside of medicine are opposed to physician-assisted dying in any form and hope that the medical profession will continue to refuse to support or participate in it. But the profession's opposition is already softening, and there is no need to look beyond our physicians for aid in dying. Many acknowledge having helped people die, and many more indicate willingness to do so, particularly if it were legal.

The extent to which physicians are already helping patients die is hard to assess. Current circumstances make it an activity to which few are willing to draw attention, not because they think that they have done wrong by their patients but because they may have done wrong by the law. Details are meager and names are usually omitted by request. Within these restrictions, twenty-four of my associates at Yale discussed their experiences and thoughts with me. Fifteen are oncologists and among the rest are specialists in neurology, pulmonary diseases, renal diseases, and AIDS—a cross-section, in short, of physicians who deal frequently with death and dying. Twenty-two had at some time been asked by a patient to shorten his or her life because of excessive suffering, and fifteen had actually done so. Most of these occasions were in the hospital through the administration of large doses of morphine, with the understanding and intention that death would be prompt. These cases obviously overlap the double effect and were often treated as precisely that. Fourteen of the physicians interviewed would vote to legalize physician-assisted dying in some form, and ten professed willingness to help patients die, either by assisted suicide or by euthanasia, if it were legal. Of those who would not do it themselves, and who might even vote against it, seven would refer patients to colleagues who felt otherwise.

Three other groups were interviewed; medical oncology fellows (postresidency trainees), fourth-year Yale medical students, and first-year medical students. The interviews took the form of small-group discussions. Six oncology fellows were evenly split in their opinions about legalizing physician-assisted dying, with two strongly in favor, two uncertain, and two strongly opposed, both for religious reasons. Only one had ever been asked by a patient for help in dying. The five fourth-year medical students had biweekly evening meetings with faculty members in my department. I assigned them two articles to read, one by Timothy Quill, recounting his own experience, and one by Leon Kass, strongly opposing physician-assisted dying.[17] I then asked them which of the two authors they would prefer as their personal physician if they had a potentially fatal illness. The discussion that ensued revealed well thought-out, unanimous opinions in favor of Quill and physician-assisted dying.

Seven first-year students met with me specifically to discuss this issue in an attempt to see whether the attitudes of the older students and young oncology residents were brought to school or acquired through exposure and discussion in school. Most of these younger students were taking an elective seminar, "The Seriously Ill Patient," given by the school chaplain, Alan Mermann, M.D., a former pediatrician. As part of their seminar, each one was assigned to follow an elderly patient who was seriously ill and could die at any time, a progressive approach to gaining an early understanding of end-of-life problems.[18] Their previous exposure to related topics laid the groundwork for an analytical discussion. Five thought that more liberal laws probably should and would be passed. More important, they thought that their attitudes largely reflected their backgrounds and premedical experiences. A much more extensive survey of the opinions of medical students, fellows, and faculty conducted at the University of Miami showed that 77 percent of students, 58 percent of residents, and 69 percent of faculty felt that there was moral justification for physicians to assist in death.[19] The concept of physician-assisted dying is clearly being given serious consideration, even by newcomers to the medical profession.

Several other polls have been conducted to assess physicians' attitudes toward assisted dying.[20] Between 20 and 50 percent of physicians contacted in the various polls had at some time received requests for assisted dying. Seven to 19 percent had provided help, assisting in suicide much more frequently than euthanasia. In most polls, however, more than 50 percent thought that assisted dying should be legalized, and almost the same number (between 40 and 53 percent) would provide assistance if it were legal. Clearly, many physicians in practice are prepared to take seriously the wishes and needs of their patients concerning death. A very influential article by ten prominent medical and legal scholars revealed that eight of them thought that "it is not immoral for a physician to assist in the rational suicide of a terminally ill person."[21] Nurses have also expressed approval of laws that would permit assisted dying.[22]

Levels of Responsibility

Responsibility for doing anything that will shorten life is shared by the patient and physician, but the actual level of responsibility for each participant differs with the several types of intervention that are possible: refusal of treatment, assisted suicide, and euthanasia.

Refusal of treatment is not technically a form of intervention at all because it is now legally accepted as a basic personal right. But the right to refuse treatment under the broadest of circumstances, as by proxy, is new and has helped to prepare the ground for our current consideration of physician-assisted dying. Several types of responsibility must be considered—psychological, causal, moral, and legal— and each differs significantly in each of these end-of-life options. Throughout this discussion we shall assume that the patient is a competent adult who personally and autonomously represents him- or herself in the discussion.

REFUSING TREATMENT

The most fundamental and widely accepted of patients' rights is the right to refuse unwanted treatment. Refusal may take place before any treatment is started, or it may take the form of a request to discontinue treatment in progress. Either way it is usually a passive strategy for both patient and physician. It carries no hint of active intervention. If nontreatment influences the time of death at all, it is usually long enough after the decision that the person can fairly be said to have died of the underlying disease and not from failure to intervene. These rational choices represent straightforward autonomy, for which the patient shoulders most of the responsibility. His right to make these decisions is widely supported by the law and now rarely poses any serious ethical or moral problem for the physician.

People with chronic renal failure who refuse dialysis and those with chronic pulmonary failure who refuse ventilatory assistance provide dramatic examples of this strategy. Both conditions involve highly technical support systems, capable of maintaining life for prolonged periods of time, but at the expense of major inconvenience and severe restrictions in lifestyle. The relation between refusal of such supportive treatment and earlier death is obvious and inescapable. A person who elects to discontinue dialysis does so with the knowledge that life will almost certainly end within one or two weeks. The decision is completely in the hands of patient and family. They need only stop the home dialysis or not show up at the hospital for scheduled appointments.

Most patients discuss their thoughts about discontinuing dialysis with the doctors and nurses involved. A nephrologist related the following example:

> We had a patient from Nigeria who was visiting his family here. He didn't feel well so they brought him to the emergency room. He turned out to have chronic renal failure. Perhaps he knew this and had been told at home that he would not be a candidate for dialysis there. We worked him up extensively, including a renal biopsy, looking for some reversible cause for his renal failure. We didn't find one so we started him on peritoneal dialysis, which was his choice. After about a year he decided to go back home, even though he knew that he could no longer get dialysis and that he would not live long. We discussed it fully, and he wanted to die with dignity at home, although he probably would have lived several years on dialysis. It was his carefully considered choice.

Discontinuing artificial respiration is a much more acute step. Death can be expected to take place within a few minutes and may be associated with serious anxiety and discomfort. Adequate sedation is essential well before the respirator is stopped to minimize these terrifying effects.[23] The moral and legal responsibility rests entirely with the patient, but turning off a ventilator represents a significant level of psychological responsibility for the physician who must do it. A colleague expressed his feelings very well: "The people making these deliberations for us have never been involved with taking people off respirators. They don't know the enormity of the act for you as a human being to end the life of another human being. It is one of those luminous experiences, when one enters a living patient's room and that living patient is part of many other people's lives, and when one exits that room, that life is no longer there. If anyone believes that a doctor can participate in that activity without experiencing some major assault on his or her own person, then one is very seriously mistaken."

The patient who is on a machine wants to end life "as it is," not life as it could be or was before the illness. He is willing to die to get away from the encumbrances required to stay alive. He realizes that discontinuing dialysis or the respirator will be fatal, which is precisely why he wants to do so. These devices are clearly artificial, and our laws sustain the point of view that they are also optional. In spite of the discomfort that disconnecting a respirator may cause the physician, the law is now strongly on the side of the competent patient who wishes to stop his treatment. The physician who is personally unwilling to accept this responsibility is obliged to find another who will.

An even more elemental step to shorten life is to discontinue artificial feeding and hydration, including feeding intravenously or via a tube directly into the stomach. Until very recently, these were considered by some to be "ordinary" supportive measures, as opposed to dialysis and ventilation, which are "extraordinary." The significance was that extraordinary measures could be refused while ordinary ones could not.[24] The courts were frequently asked to intervene, and now they usually do not distinguish between extraordinary and ordinary measures of life support.

A variant of refusing or discontinuing artificial feeding occurs when a person simply decides not to eat, forgoing all food and drink for the week or more that it takes to die, typically of dehydration.[25] Many cancers, including most of those originating in the gastrointestinal tract, eventually cause death by starvation and dehydration. Fortunately, the suffering associated with starvation is moderated significantly by the extreme weakness and clouded senses associated with the terminal disease.[26] The person who invites such a death at an earlier time may be using an inevitable mechanism to shorten his life. It should be noted that an early death from dehydration is not a natural death from the underlying disease but rather from the patient's active choice. Still, there is no legal or moral proscription in current thinking against a physician's adequately medicating a person who elects starvation. The patient may be deliberately shortening his or her own life—technically committing suicide—but the physician is only providing comfort. The proverbial discomfort of starvation and dehydration discourage most people from even considering this way out. But for some who will eventually die this way anyway, an earlier death by starvation may be an acceptable compromise.

A woman whom I interviewed and followed had two sources of severe pain, debilitating arthritis and advanced breast cancer with bone metastasis. She discussed help in dying with her very attentive and sympathetic internist. He told her that he could not go that far, but she secretly hoped that he would. Failing that, she had two daughters who promised to help if her situation became unbearable. She was certain that she would not take her own life but sincerely hoped that someone would help if she needed it. Her problem was fairly typical:

> I'm eighty-one years old, and until recently I could do everything. Now I can hardly even cook and feed myself. The pain is exhausting, night and day. I am a doer, not a sitter, and I get very depressed. The loneliness and the pain and helplessness are getting worse and have made me think of suicide many times. I have lots of friends, but I am still very much alone. I have a wonderful doctor and I have been on every antidepressant there is—no help. But I just couldn't do it myself. If I take sleeping pills, I may make myself worse. I thought of turning on the car in the garage, but it was winter and I said, "I can't possibly do that. It's too cold out there. I'll wait for the summer." I have lots of morphine in the house, but I'm just afraid to do it by myself. When it gets bad enough, I'll call my daughters or my doctor or something.

About a year later, when her condition had deteriorated as expected, she decided that the time had come. Again her doctor, who was now coming to her home several times a week, said that he would continue to help in any way he could but that he could not give her a lethal injection. She was now dependent on outside help from home hospice, visiting nurses, and housekeepers. Her daughters understood that with so many nonfamily people in the house, it would be risky for them to do anything to shorten their mother's life. At this point the woman announced her own solution: she was going to stop eating and drinking. She asked her daughters to make a nice dinner of her favorite foods; they shared what she had decided would be her last meal. Her bed was now in a corner of the dining room, and she insisted that her daughters eat there so that they could talk together. In a few days she became so weak that she could no longer get out of bed, but she seemed at peace with her decision, even with food close at hand. Her doctor helped by providing her with medication patches that eliminated most of her sensations of hunger and thirst. Several days after she began her fast she died.

PHYSICIAN-ASSISTED SUICIDE

Life-shortening measures that are based on the patient's right to refuse treatment are legal in most states. With the exception of discontinuing treatment by actively turning off a respirator, the physician functions primarily in an advisory and supportive capacity. But physician-assisted dying, including assisted suicide and euthanasia, is illegal in most states. The purpose is the same—relief of suffering, albeit at the cost of life itself. But in providing any form of personal assistance, the physician assumes an increasingly central and active role, psychologically, morally, and legally.

A physician who has agreed to assist in a patient's suicide usually provides a prescription for a sleeping medication that suppresses respiration when taken in large doses. Barbiturates are the most commonly used drugs.[27] Because large doses can cause vomiting, an antiemetic is often taken first. More complex devices, such as Kevorkian's suicide machine or his use of carbon monoxide, require that the system be set up by the doctor. For the death to remain technical suicide, however, any device must ultimately be activated by the patient.[28] Moral responsibility is shared by the physician who provides the prescription and the patient who ingests the drugs. Although in theory a patient's judgment could be impaired or he could be coerced into suicide by someone else, his ostensible freedom to perform or retreat from the fatal act is strong evidence of volition.

Many physicians prefer the idea of giving a prescription precisely because they do not want to be present at the time of death. Time provides distance for the physician, who may find comfort in the fact that the eventual death is remote from the day she wrote the prescription. If the interval is sufficiently long, she may only suspect that the drugs were taken and may be able to believe that death resulted from the disease. Physician-assisted suicide can now be done most safely when it involves very few people and can be made to look like a natural death, allowing the physician to sign the death certificate accordingly and avoid questions.

The physician may also deceive herself. Even though the patient wants to die, the physician can convince herself that the pills have really been requested for sleep, further reducing the doctor's responsibility for what the patient does with them. An oncologist presented this rationale:

A patient who had terminal cancer asked for sleeping medicines because he was having trouble sleeping. He gave me the message, indirectly but clearly, that his intent was to eventually use that medication to end his life. I told him that if he needed the medications to help him sleep, I would be able and willing to give them to him. I wanted to make it clear that that was the sole reason that I would be willing to give him the medicine. Then I asked him if that was the reason he was going to use it, and he said it was. I continued giving him the medications, and about two weeks later he died in his sleep. I suspect that he took all the medication, but I don't know for sure. Now you might say that I was asking my patient to be dishonest. Suppose a patient was honest and said to me, "No doc, that's not the reason I'm going to use the medicine. Life's unbearable, and I want to use the medicine you're prescribing for me to end my life." I personally would not be able to prescribe the medicine to him if he made it that explicit, because that's not the reason I prescribe sleeping medicine.

Some physicians are bothered specifically by their lack of control. The patient who wants sleeping pills to have on hand "just in case" may feel great relief in knowing that he has the means to end his suffering when and if he wants to. Another person, on the other hand, may have a temporary setback in his disease and decide irrationally that "just in case" is now, long before it needs to be, and for entirely the wrong reasons. Unless the patient brings it up, the physician is not apt to have an opportunity to influence the decision. For this reason there may be situations where the physician feels that she should be the gatekeeper and not provide the patient with the means until the disease is sufficiently advanced and all treatment options have been used up or refused. Obviously, the physician retains control until she gives the patient the prescription for the drugs. An oncologist described a patient who was psychologically very erratic:

> She had melanoma, and when she was doing well she was the happiest, most functional person you can imagine. But when she was ill, from her tumor or from chemotherapy, she was profoundly depressed. The psychiatrist said he could not do very much because she was appropriately depressed. I sent her to a support group which she almost ruined—she drained everybody in the group. She asked me if I would give her some "strong" sleeping pills to have on hand. I said I would, but that I would hold off until she was really at the end of the road. Right now she is fine, with no known tumor at all, but a little bad news completely upsets her. It has happened before so I will be very careful about when I give her the medicine she wants.

Medical progress has made the use of sleeping pills for physician-assisted suicide more complicated. For many years barbiturates, primarily Seconal and Phenobarbital, were the most widely used hypnotics. The side effect of overdosage is respiratory depression, and deliberate overdosage was a common way for people to take their own lives. Today, these drugs have been largely replaced by equally effective hypnotics—Dalmane, Halcyon, Restoril, Ambien, and others—which do not have this side effect. To obtain barbiturates the patient must either explain his reason and ask the physician for them outright or accept the other drugs but complain to the physician that they did not help him sleep and that he needs something stronger. The physician may prescribe a barbiturate without further questioning, perhaps recognizing the true purpose but without having to acknowledge it. She may also flatly refuse when she does recognize the purpose. Even if the drugs are prescribed, the infrequent use of barbiturates as hypnotics might cause a pharmacist to question the prescription. A large pharmacy contacted in this study reported filling prescriptions for Seconal only two or three times a year. Barbiturates are also readily available "on the street," but the patient must have an illegal connection to get them from this source.

VOLUNTARY ACTIVE EUTHANASIA

The ultimate step in physician-assisted dying is voluntary euthanasia. In Holland this is usually done with an intravenous injection of a barbiturate to induce deep sleep, followed by an injection of a muscle relaxant to stop respiration.[29] Death ensues in a few minutes. Both physician-assisted suicide and euthanasia stem from the desire of patients to have more control over how their lives end. In physician-assisted suicide the patient assumes full control once he has been provided with the means. In euthanasia the patient gives up some control in order to have reliable and responsible help. He still shares in the moral responsibility and must request the help and make the final decision. At the last instant, however, he must relinquish control to his physician. The cancer patient who wishes to lessen his suffering may either do so earlier, while he can still take the necessary pills, or rely on his physician to keep her word that she will do it for him when he cannot. The former means losing an unspecified quantity of life that still retains some quality, while the latter allows extending life to the limit of endurance. Just the promise of the physician to help at the end might encourage a person to live longer and enjoy the twilight of life fully, secure in the knowledge that death will be humane, painless, and still under his control.

I think that voluntary active euthanasia eventually should be included under the legal mantle of assisted dying. The first laws to be passed in most states will undoubtedly be limited to assisted suicide. Although this seems less radical to lawmakers and less personal to physicians, it will place a tremendous burden on some patients. If we focus our medical and legal attention on the patient's condition and wishes, it will be clear that the method of assisted dying is secondary and should include euthanasia. Indeed, some physicians may even prefer to have greater responsibility right from the beginning, knowing that if they had greater control there would be little or no chance of failure. Undoubtedly many patients would prefer just that.

If euthanasia were legal, the main prerequisite would be a trusting relationship with a physician who was willing to step in when called upon. The terms of the partnership should be negotiated at the beginning rather than the end. The physician who could not enter into such a partnership would be expected to make her position clear when the issue first came up and to help the patient find another physician who felt differently. The patient must be free to reconsider at any time, but the physician who has agreed to help should not withdraw at the last minute.

In deliberately bringing about a "good death" through voluntary euthanasia, the physician assumes a far greater personal role than in physician-assisted suicide, one that is unmistakably active. She gives the drugs herself. If she does so with the intent of helping the patient die, there is no way of hiding behind the ethical and moral uncertainties of a double effect. Nor can the timing soften the issue: the doctor injects the drug, and within a few minutes death occurs. She understands and respects the patient's wish to end his suffering. Indeed, her relationship with her patient must be such that she feels a responsibility that exceeds her discomfort in participating in the death of a human being. The emotional cost of this was described to me by a doctor in Holland: "Whenever I help someone to die, I usually end up sitting on the edge of the bed with a member of the family, crying together. When suffering is so great that a person asks for death, it is better for the doctor to have to cry a little than for the patient and the family to cry alone. After that I find I have to be by myself quite a lot. For a few days I am not good company. I don't find it easy to help people die."

A complicated and controversial procedure related to voluntary euthanasia is nonvoluntary euthanasia, in which a noncompetent patient's life is terminated, at the instigation of a third party, whether family member, physician, or other proxy. The background for this, the patient who is in coma and unable to comprehend or respond at all, has been the subject of several court decisions. The courts have allowed third parties, typically family, to authorize withdrawal of such basic life-sustaining measures as artificial respiration and even nutrition. This is not considered to be euthanasia, and more active intervention is usually unnecessary because death occurs when all artificial aid is removed.

Far more complicated and more accurately described as nonvoluntary euthanasia is the circumstance of a patient who is conscious but demented and therefore unable to understand his condition or options. Society has an obligation to protect the lives of such people from being jeopardized by family, caregivers, or even the exertion by society itself of financial pressure. These patients are potential victims of abuse. They are also potential victims of severe suffering and pointless prolongation of life. The most obvious example, as we have seen, may be the Alzheimer's patient who is totally incompetent but who, at a time when he was well and fully able to make such a decision, made clear his wishes not to be kept alive in a demented state.

Finally, the true opposite of voluntary euthanasia is involuntary euthanasia, in which a patient is competent and wishes to live but some other authority—family, caregiver, or state—overrides his wishes and insists that he be put to death. Aside from cases of capital punishment—itself a morally ambiguous practice—this ultimate assertion of power is classified as murder.

Assisted Suicide Versus Euthanasia

Across the spectrum of patient-physician interactions to shorten life, the law in most of the United States permits no physician-assisted dying, neither suicide nor euthanasia. Comparing these remains hypothetical. The legal and moral boundaries are shifting, however, and the similarities and differences between assisted suicide and euthanasia should be clearly understood. Even now our laws look upon these two actions very differently. Neither is usually prosecuted, particularly when carried out by a physician at the request of the dying patient. But assisted suicide is a much lesser crime, punishable by a fine or brief imprisonment; in some jurisdictions it is not a crime at all. Euthanasia is considered to be a form of manslaughter or even murder, punishable by a long imprisonment or even death.

The main reasons for patients to request assistance in dying are physical or psychological inability to do it alone and fear of failure. These reasons apply differently to assisted suicide and euthanasia. Inability to do it alone ranges from difficulty obtaining drugs to a need for assistance in ingesting the drugs. Many patients express unwillingness to do it alone even though they are physically able. Even the presence of the physician at the time of death from assisted suicide might not satisfy the wish to have someone else assume or at least share the ultimate responsibility. This concern may reflect abhorrence of taking one's own life or ambivalence about early death, or simply an understandable desire to transfer to someone else such an awesome task. Euthanasia might be the choice of a person who questions his own resolve. Euthanasia might also be preferred by some who would take their own lives if need be, if their suffering were great enough and suicide the only option.

Another important distinction between assisted suicide and euthanasia is the opportunity for a person to change his mind at the last minute. Ambivalence is an almost universal component of any decision about shortening life. Opening the door to the physician who is prepared to give a lethal injection must seem to some like closing the door on further procrastination or negotiation. The presence of the physician at assisted suicide might have the same effect.[30] Even the presence of close family members might formalize the event to a point where the patient feels that he cannot renege. To counteract these perceived pressures it is essential that the patient be reassured repeatedly by physician and family that there is no contract to be broken, that he may change his mind at any time.[31]

ACTIVE AND PASSIVE EUTHANASIA

A confusing pair of terms, active and passive euthanasia are too deeply ingrained in our literature to be avoided. As early as 1884 it was argued that "perhaps logically it is difficult to justify a passive more than an active attempt at euthanasia; but certainly it is less abhorrent to our feelings. To surrender to superior forces is not the same thing as to lead the attack of the enemy upon one's friends. May there not come a time when it is a duty in the interest of the survivors to stop a fight which is only prolonging a useless and hopeless struggle."[32] In the sequence of interventions we have examined, assisted suicide and euthanasia are both classified as active euthanasia by some, because some degree of physician participation is required in both. Others label as active only those interventions in which the physician personally administers the drug. Passive euthanasia includes withholding or withdrawing treatment by request of a patient whose intent is to end his life.

Although the need for a category of passive euthanasia has been lessened by the establishment of the legal right of a person to refuse unwanted treatment, the concept remains alive in the minds of many ethicists because it has been used to set a boundary between what was deemed morally permissible and what was not. Most Western religions have adopted this distinction, as has the law. The moral ground is shifting, though, and many people have medical conditions for which assisted dying seems reasonable and acceptable, but they have no life support systems that can be withdrawn. As the moral similarity between these situations becomes accepted, the law must address the shifts in society's moral values.[33]

"Passive" euthanasia is really a misnomer. We have already seen that some activities that are acceptable, like discontinuing a respirator, are not psychologically passive for the responsible physician. Euthanasia embodies the spirit of being helped to die rather than being allowed to die. It is also strange to speak of euthanasia on the one hand while denying on the other that death is intended at all. Death is central in both intent and result. Indeed, intent is the main weakness in the concept of passive euthanasia. Many activities are deemed acceptable as long as the primary purpose is relief of suffering. That death may follow immediately is not the issue, as long as it is not the original goal. We can see, then, that intent is defined by the speaker, with little reference to the act or result. The language is softened by adding *passive,* the act is assuaged by allowing the patient to die, however long it may take, and intent is left up to the imagination of the patient and the honesty of the physician. The result, though, is early death. If the reason for passive steps is the relief of suffering but the result is death, why should the concept not be extended to physician-assisted dying, including active euthanasia, for the same reason and with the same result?

Some ethicists feel that there is no significant moral difference between letting a person die and helping a person to die. In allowing death to take place, control is relinquished to nature and the time of death is determined by the disease. Some eagerly desired deaths may even have to wait for the occurrence of an acute illness, usually a chance infection, for which treatment can be withheld. Or worse, "a patient who otherwise might have preferred to go on living a bit longer may feel pressured to take advantage of today's opportunity to refuse treatment rather than chance the fact that such a 'window of opportunity' may not return in a timely fashion in the future."[34] The medical ethicist James Rachels has pointed out that withholding treatment from a near-terminal patient to "allow" him to have a slow and painful demise may be less humane than assisting in his death. "Once the initial decision not to prolong his agony has been made, active euthanasia is actually preferable to passive euthanasia, rather than the reverse. To say otherwise is to endorse the option that leads to more suffering rather than less."[35]

It seems inconsistent to permit a patient to refuse treatment that may prolong life but to refuse a request for assisted dying under similar circumstances. As we have seen, for some illnesses, there are no machines, no life-sustaining switch to turn off, however great the need. Recently the courts have begun to agree with this line of thinking. In 1996 the Court of Appeals for the Second Circuit declared the laws against physician-assisted dying of New York, Connecticut, and Vermont to be unconstitutional on the grounds of equal protection.[36] Its reasoning was that because terminally ill patients have the right to hasten death by asking that treatment be stopped, similar patients should also have the right to hasten death by asking a physician to actually administer certain drugs. The U.S. Supreme Court did not agree with this reasoning, sustaining a perceived difference between active and passive euthanasia.

DOUBLE EFFECT

Medicine has a commonly used back door to euthanasia. The double effect is often invoked to justify the use of large doses of morphine to relieve pain in cancer, while recognizing that such doses will suppress respiration and may hasten death. The principle of double effect affirms that as long as the primary intent is to relieve pain, the secondary result is acceptable. This concept was first codified by St. Thomas Aquinas to rationalize killing in self-defense and in war, in the face of the church's strong stand against any killing of human be ings. Killing under these circumstances is secondary to the main intent, which is to save one's own life. The good effect is that I will live, the unfortunate but foreseen bad effect is that my attacker will die.

Adapted to purely medical circumstances, the double effect has four requirements:

1. The drug must be given primarily for its good effect, namely, to relieve pain.
2. The bad effect, death, must not be required in order to relieve pain.
3. Death should not be the intended result of giving the drug but may be foreseen and accepted as a possible consequence thereof.
4. The benefit to the patient in relief of pain should outweigh the risk of harm, namely, earlier death.[37]

The concept of double effect, based as it is on primary intent, has satisfied our religious and moral needs for centuries and may even grow in importance now. Because intent can be nebulous and sub jective and can be adjusted to meet the circumstances, however, the law finds the double effect less useful. The law is more concerned with the results of an action than it is with the intent. Personal intentions are hard to prove or disprove, and rarely if ever would a physician's sole intent be to kill a patient without some preponderant background reason, such as to relieve suffering. Relief of pain by the use of large doses of narcotics is widely accepted, and the question is how far can the physician go in providing such relief before intent is questioned and the bounds of the double effect exceeded?[38] From the point of view of the patient who sees death as preferable to continued suffering, death may indeed be his primary, not secondary, goal. In the current legal climate, where the physician is squeezed between the demands to provide compassionate relief and laws against assisted dying that are never enforced, we can expect the double effect to be used and cited increasingly frequently to help physicians, patients, and society itself solve a difficult problem.

Toward the end of life narcotics are often given continuously, as a morphine drip. The doses are rarely reduced as death approaches and pain sensation decreases. The patient is rendered insensate by the drugs, relieved of pain and apprehension of death but also left unable to formulate or communicate his own wishes. Indeed, complete control has been assumed by the physician. More important, the primary and secondary effects of the drugs are often reversed, even in the mind of the physician. A medical oncologist explained this predicament:

> "Euthanasia is practiced in the hospital, and it's practiced at
> hospices. Do people think that every time morphine is given,
> it is because the patient has requested a shot for pain? The an-
> swer is no! In oncology, we help patients end their lives all the
> time by using morphine drips and increasing the dose, osten-
> sibly to control their pain but knowing full well that at a high
> enough dose we are likely to stop respiration. I explain to the
> family: if the patient stops breathing, and that may happen
> with this medication, we probably should not do anything to
> intervene. Everybody generally nods their head yes and says,
> "Just try to keep him comfortable," and that's the end of the
> discussion. Nobody asks, "Are you really saying that you are
> going to help him die?" It's obvious what we are doing. We
> just say it a bit more gracefully. It is better that certain aspects
> of this are unstated. When things are bad enough, we often
> help anyway, even if it is not requested. The morphine drip is
> frequently a one-way street, and I don't think that anybody
> should pretend otherwise. But it is a medically and socially ac-
> ceptable way for the physician to assist at the end of life.

Oncologists make such frequent use of the double effect of narcotics that some see little need for new laws that would more formally permit physician-assisted dying. Many of them prefer the unstructured and unsupervised status quo to any change that might require more open discussion and reporting, or at least recording their activities. A physician in Seattle pointed out the inconsistency of our present position: "When physicians secretly and silently adapt a normal medical practice to hasten dying, we are on shaky ground indeed if we say that they may not do so openly and honestly."[39]

The extreme use of narcotics to relieve pain at the end of life is terminal sedation. The patient requests enough sedation to be maintained in coma, and food and fluids are no longer given. This is at the very edge of the double effect because it is usually done at the patient's request and with the obvious intent that death will be painless and certain.[40] It should be recognized, however, that the use of large doses of narcotics in people who are dying can be very close to euthanasia, dressed up for social acceptability.[41] Furthermore, it may resemble voluntary, nonvoluntary, or even involuntary euthanasia, depending on who initiates the process. Euthanasia and double effect in this situation are separated only by intent. If the drugs are given primarily to relieve pain, earlier death is accepted as the result of the double-effect. But if the primary intent is indeed to shorten life, the act is euthanasia, and sometimes even involuntary euthanasia. Physicians take real liberties with what they consider to be best for their patients and what they think their patients would want, even though the patients may not have been asked. Thus the acceptable practice of the double effect borders on the most questionable practice of involuntary euthanasia.

The possibility of using the double effect of narcotics to bring about an earlier and more comfortable death is limited to diseases such as cancer and AIDS and respiratory failure, where discomfort and pain are normally treated with these drugs. This is unfair to people with other very distressing illnesses, primarily neurological diseases such as multiple sclerosis and amyotrophic lateral sclerosis, who are also entitled to have an end to their suffering. Narcotics do not feature prominently in the treatment of these diseases, so their use to shorten life under the guise of the double effect can be difficult or inappropriate.

The need to have a moral and legal loophole by which physicians can help patients die has led some to overemphasize the double effect and even to assume that any time enough narcotic is given to control severe pain, life is automatically shortened. The result is that physicians may again become fearful of giving enough medication. Now their concern is not addiction, as it was in the past, but possible accusations of having assisted the patient to die. When the stigma of assisted dying is removed, this will not be an issue. Until then, the vagaries of intent and double effect should never be allowed to interfere with compassionate care in relieving pain.

For our mother and our family, it was a good way because there was plenty of time to say goodbye. Not a moment, not a day since she died have we been sorry for how her life ended. We know that she comes back once in a while, and when she does she tells us that it was a very nice way to die, and that it was the right thing to do.

A young woman describing her mother's assisted death

4 Dying Alone or Dying with Help:

Our Frightened Society

Our culture in the United States, and indeed in most of the Western world, is oriented toward youth. The increasing number of aged in the population is often seen as a social embarrassment, a political problem, and a financial liability. The culmination of old age and illness is death, and our society fears death. Strong pressures discourage the individual from thinking about death, and certainly from talking about it. Although some forethought is forced on us by family and financial needs, planning for death in more direct and personal ways remains rare. Life insurance is purchased to safeguard spouses and provide for education, even to pay taxes. Wills are written to ensure the desired distribution of property. But these arrangements are usually carried out in good health, years in advance; death is remote and abstract.

The ability to plan the specifics of one's own death was enhanced by the advent of several forms of advance directives and the legal recognition of a patient's right of self-determination, even to the extent of being able to refuse treatment. As we shall see, advance directives are still not widely used, and very few patients have life-support systems that can be discontinued if they wish. Planning the actual event, as a potentially active participant, is usually considered morbid, abnormal behavior. Society says that one must be diverted and distracted from this mode of thought, however realistic it may be. "You shouldn't think that way," say family members—and, with remarkable frequency, health care professionals—even when illness is far advanced and there is no other logical way to think.

The veil of avoidance with which our society surrounds death isolates its victim. He may suffer in silence or say what he wants, but no one seems to listen. Even physicians have been known to shun their dying patients. And laws make it impossible to carry out the most reasoned of plans for confronting death in a positive fashion if such plans require outside help. This kind of avoidance clearly serves only to artificially insulate victim and society as a whole from an unpleasant reality. Many people would like at least the possibility of assistance in dying. Ideally, planning for death would include patient, family, clergy, if desired, and physician. The act would take place in a location of choice, usually at home, and the physician's participation would be within the law.

The Netherlands is experimenting with just such a framework and has become a social laboratory in which assisted dying can be examined in all of its varieties and implications. To evaluate the relevance of the Dutch experience, we contrast a death in Holland with one in the United States, where assisted death is still seen by many as a very dangerous issue.

Suicide Today

Under our current laws, suicide is often a violent, lonely, antisocial act. The intelligent person usually realizes that thoughts of suicide must be private and that the planning is best carried out in total secrecy. Even a verbal clue of such disquieting ideas to physician, family, or friends can lead to discovery and thence to failure. The hidden gun or the pills will be searched for and almost certainly found, and any modicum of privacy will be denied. After the planning, the act itself must also be carried out secretly. The risk now is not only discovery and failure but responsibility for the safety of others, for whom any element of participation is forbidden by law. Because of this, any emotional sharing of the experience of death—any opportunity to say good-bye—is out of the question. Compassion is risky. As if the disease itself had not forced its own share of isolation and loneliness through loss of activity and inability to see friends, the contemplated suicide draws the curtain on a drama that is still very much in progress. There is no opportunity to question the wisdom of the act, to discuss it in a meaningful fashion with anyone, or to obtain the desired permission to sever lifelong relationships so arbitrarily. This inability to share the experience breeds enormous guilt that cannot be buffered by any form of human kindness. A person who loves his family but must plan his death in secret usually realizes what pain his action is going to engender. He is under great pressure to talk to them, to reassure them that his act is an escape from his disease and not a rejection of his family, but he is unable to do so. The act itself is usually terrifying and terrible. One wonders how many desperately ill patients do *not* take their own lives, suffering to the end to protect their families from the trauma and stigma associated with a typical suicide. Certain death often requires violence at a time when one has already been damaged by disease and would prefer a peaceful and dignified end over further destruction and disfigurement.

After the death comes further distress for the family. As one author has commented, "Suicide is the skeleton left by the deceased in the survivor's closet."[1] The horrible surprise, the visual image of the dead loved one, the overwhelming guilt of not having recognized the problem and done something about it, the sense of rejection from the secret planning, and the realization that the person died in the absence of love and caring—all these perceptions combine to make the final loss far more devastating than it would have been had it resulted from the disease itself. The violent implication of rejection that suicide expresses to the family can be catastrophic. Every personal or financial disagreement, every missed opportunity to talk together and express gratitude and forgiveness, every pressure to accept or conform becomes a source of guilt. The acute guilt must die of its own exhaustion, for it cannot be explored and resolved with the single most important party. In fact, the family's burden of guilt and shame may never completely disappear; sometimes, those feelings are instead pushed into the recesses of the unconscious, where they may lie hidden and internalized, often festering to the point of causing their own serious psychological problems over the years. The stigma of suicide, though less than it once was, still hangs heavily in our society; the family of the suicide is poisoned, too.

Much of the collateral trauma of suicide occurs whether or not the attempt is successful. But a failed attempt also carries its own curse. At one of our weekly medical conferences we discussed a patient who had tried unsuccessfully to kill himself. Joseph was sixty years old when he was found to have inoperable lung cancer. He began chemotherapy with the understanding that the treatment could prolong his life for a few months but could not possibly cure him. The combination of the disease and his treatment put severe restrictions on his life. He rarely left the house and no longer wanted to see people. In spite of strong medication, his pain was constant and relentless, and he could not force his mind to focus on much else. He began to wonder why he was going through all this for a few extra months of misery. He discussed his mounting concerns several times with his doctor, who never denied that the cancer was progressing and that he could expect no more than a few more months. His pain medication was increased, but his doctor politely brushed aside questions about whether an earlier death might not be better than prolonged suffering. After one of these discussions, when his family was out of the house for the day, he bought a gun. It remained in his bedside drawer for two and a half months.

At his last weekly visit with his oncologist Joe began to cry and said that he did not know how much longer he could endure. He asked for some pills that he could keep on hand to use to end his life if his illness and pain became unendurable. The doctor explained that he would do everything in his power to provide comfort but that it would be against the law to provide drugs to facilitate suicide. He explained that physicians are educated to help people live rather than to help them die, and he went on to review the pain medications and increased them considerably. He also arranged for Joe to come to the hospital the next day for a blood transfusion that would increase his strength.

Joe was furious. He felt angry and abandoned. He had asked for real help and was given a condescending pat on the head. Worse than the pain, which was bad enough, he was dying by inches, shedding more weight every week, even though he already seemed to be nothing but skin and bones. He didn't want more pain medication, and he had no use for more strength. He just wanted it all to end, as soon as possible, and he wanted someone to see it his way and give him some help.

When they parted, he asked the doctor not to discuss the conversation with his wife or family. He had always been afraid of being in the hospital, and he did not come in for the blood transfusion. That evening, while his wife was cooking dinner, he shot himself in the abdomen. His wife rushed upstairs to find him conscious but bleeding. She dialed 911.

In the emergency room, the last thing he said before being intubated was that "I have lung cancer and I'm dying. I don't want to live." The tube then cut off all communication. An operation was deemed mandatory, and his wife signed the permission for it. The bullet was found to have injured the stomach, the colon, and the spleen, all reparable injuries.

While Joe was in the operating room, his wife, son, and daughter-in-law cross-examined each other. Where had he gotten the gun? He hated even the idea of guns and had never had one in the house before. They couldn't believe that he felt desperate enough to plan such a violent end for himself. His wife began to have her own disquieting questions. What could she have done to prevent it? What had she done to cause it? Joe's medical oncologist explained the extent of the disease, and they all agreed to allow him to forgo resuscitation if he survived the surgery.

He did survive. When his family next saw him, he was lying peacefully in bed, fully conscious and extremely unhappy. A woman was sitting outside the door of his room. He would have to have a guard outside his room at all times, and the psychiatric team would examine him and recommend appropriate treatment. His wife was shocked. "He's not a mental case, he's not a criminal, he's dying of cancer. That's why he did this."

The oncologist described Joe as an independent person who was depressed by his illness, though he had no history of depression. Joe had refused even to consider repeated suggestions that he see a psychiatrist for the depression. On the other hand, the doctor characterized Joe as a gentle, nonviolent man and said that he was surprised by what had happened: "The idea that he might use a gun on himself was something which just never occurred to me."

Joe's wife wanted to ask him many things—in particular, why he had done it. But she couldn't. She rarely knew what he was thinking, and she knew that she wouldn't find out now. Instead, she sat in the chair at his bedside for two days, dozing at night. On the third day he died quietly.

Several lessons can be drawn from this unfortunate episode. Dialing 911 activates a system that is almost impossible to turn off. The paramedics have limited and well-defined responsibilities, and the primary function of the emergency room is the saving of life. The director of emergency services at Yale–New Haven Hospital claims that a person who attempts suicide by overdosing on drugs has a less than one in five hundred chance of succeeding if he or she arrives in the emergency room alive. A person with a gunshot wound that is not immediately fatal also has a very reasonable chance of surviving if surgery is performed promptly.

Halting emergency treatment once the patient has arrived in the hospital is exceedingly difficult. It requires that the medical status of the patient be completely understood and confirmed by the patient's own physician, usually in person. It also requires that the patient and family all agree—even insist—that no treatment be carried out. The family must be comfortable with the decision, for they are the ones who will have to live with it. Given the unexpected nature of the incident and the time constraints in the emergency room, these conditions are rarely met. The hospital also has an obligation to provide a protective environment for the suicidal patient to prevent further attempts at self-injury. This requires that the patient be monitored, occasionally even sedated or restrained, for as long as necessary. These precautions are necessary to give the hospital and its physicians and nurses legal protection, as well as to safeguard the life of the patient.

An emergency physician explained the prevailing attitude in his department:

> We seem to have a special block when it comes to suicide. When a patient who is known to be terminally ill comes in with severe pneumonia or has been in an automobile accident, and all signs say "do not resuscitate," we stand back. However, when the same patient with a terminal illness takes matters into his own hands by injuring himself, or taking an overdose of medication, we are not comfortable with letting him go ahead and die. We find every possible reason to intervene. Unfortunately, we still consider attempted suicide to be a sign of mental illness, and when it fails, the person is turned over to the psychiatric service, no matter what the circumstances.

An Assisted Death

In a legally assisted death, the dreadful need for dying alone, abhorrent to patient and family alike, is eliminated. The death can take place in a location of maximum comfort and security, usually at home, with familiar surroundings and loved ones present. It need not be a lonely, secret event. The physician can offer to be present, if the patient wishes to have her there. A minister, priest, or rabbi can be included on the same basis. With physician assistance, death is not a violent destruction and desecration but comes as gently and peacefully as sleep. Fear of discovery and failure are eliminated. The timing can be set so that family members can be there, from however far away, a condition that is often impossible in hospitals or nursing homes, or indeed in any unplanned death.

I met with the family of Margke Vegter in their home near Rotterdam, the house where she died by euthanasia eight months before. About 80 percent of assisted deaths in the Netherlands are for cancer, and Margke had advanced breast cancer. Her husband, Dick, is about fifty and works as a freelance filmmaker. Xandra, their daughter, is twenty-three, has her own work and lives away from home. Elderick, their son, and Nadine, their second daughter, twenty-two and nineteen respectively, are students and live at home with their father. It is obviously a very close family. Margke's illness was a responsibility for the entire family, as was her death. I was surprised and pleased that they wished to meet with me as a family, too. They started by showing me a portrait photo on the living room wall of a beautiful, lively, smiling woman, their wife and mother, who had died so recently. Although I will relate Mrs. Vegter's story mostly through one voice, her husband's, all four shared in the telling.

"Five years ago my wife found a small lump in her breast," Dick Vegter told me.

> The family doctor did not think it was serious but that it should be biopsied. We were told right away that the biopsy was positive and that an operation would be necessary. Two

lymph nodes were involved, and it clearly was not a very good situation. Things went well for a while, and we had good times, but then the cancer came back in the very same area, and she had to have another operation.

After the surgery she had chemotherapy and also radiation. She really had everything that was possible at that time, including Taxol. In the beginning she said, "I'm going to go for it," and later she could honestly say that she had done everything possible to hold back her disease and get more time. But the battle against cancer is hard, and eventually she realized that she was not going to win. The problem was that the cancer kept coming back, always in the same area. Later it spread to her spine, and then she was found to have a shadow in her lung, which also turned out to be a tumor. The longest time span that we did not visit the hospital was three months. Over all those years, we lived on hope and prayer.

Early in her illness she had heard about the possible consequences of her kind of cancer, and she was already thinking about how it could end. She had a very positive but very realistic attitude: "When the time comes, it will end. Until then, I will enjoy my life. My children are here and I have had a very nice life. I have a wonderful husband, I have a house, I have my work. I'm going to live as long as I want, but not longer." She brought up the thought of euthanasia herself five years before she died, when she first found out that she had this cancer. We all felt that it was her decision and that if it seemed like the right thing to do when the time came, we would agree with her.

The time to make this kind of decision is in a good moment, when you are feeling well and are able to plan ahead clearly. At first you hope that the cancer can be cured, but after a while you realize that it cannot and the doctor confirms this. But she was never depressed about the situation. We thought that when she went upstairs she would be angry and crying. But then we found out that she was not angry at all. She was reading her books. She was very optimistic and sometimes even made jokes about it. We thought that she should be depressed and that her behavior was not normal, but it continued year after year, right to the end. For her it was definitely normal. I think this was because she had accepted the fact that she was ill.

The family doctor is the first line in Holland. The second line is the specialist. She had three specialists, a radiation therapist, a medical oncologist, and Dr. van Eych, her surgeon. She was closest to Dr. van Eych and had already asked him to organize her care with the others. He had known her for five years and she had complete trust in him. He was helpful throughout every aspect of her illness. He was also very helpful to us and explained everything to us many times. He came to the house the day that she died and was here throughout the evening.

All her friends knew what she planned to do, and there were lots of them. Many came to visit her and say goodbye in the last weeks. None of the friends tried to talk her out of her plan. There was no secret about it. People could always ask us how she was doing, and we would tell them. After she died friends were not afraid to come into the house, even though somebody had died upstairs. They were glad to see us and we were glad to see them.

At the end of 1994 we visited Morocco, and while we were there she said she thought it had come back again. We would see the doctor as soon as we got home, after the New Year, but she said not to tell the children or anyone else until after the holidays. She seemed to know that this might be the last time. She had already had all the treatments possible. She realized that every time it came back her medical possibilities were smaller, and again smaller, and perhaps now none at all. By March the lymphatics were blocked up in her arm and she

had amazing swelling, which was very painful. She again began to talk about how things were going with her and what
the future was. Every time we talked about it she said, "Well, I
will know when the time comes, and I'm not going all the way
to the end. There will be no machines and no morphine to the
maximum. I came into the world as a baby but I'm not going
to leave it that way." Then we discussed what we would do.
We discussed whether she would prefer to be in the hospital
or at home, knowing that she could have help in dying in either place. Her choice was to be at home.

In the last few weeks she was confined to her bed and we
had help come in to take care of her. We had visiting nurses,
but we did everything around the house; we cleaned the room
and did the cooking and took very good care of her. It was terrible for her that we had to help her to go to the toilet and to
do every little thing. For us it was all right. If someone is sick,
you help. But for her, she was the mother, and still a young
mother. Normally she helped us and she thought it was very
bad that we had to help her. She thought her illness was too
much of a strain for us. We told her that that was not a good
reason at all. We were doing just fine. The only reasons to end
her life would have to be for medical reasons.

Earlier we had a hard time talking about some things, but
when the decision was finally made, it was a change for everyone. Then we could talk and laugh and love each other like a
real family. During this time we talked with her about *everything*. Very long, very deep conversations. Afterward we
would think we had nothing left to say—we had covered
everything. It's important to be able to talk about your life together, the lives of your children, what's behind them, and
what's ahead of them. Strangely, in the final days, there was
humor in our talk. We could laugh about things together right
to the very last day.

It helped her to have the decision made so that she knew

that at any time she could say "All right, that is it." But she also wanted to hear from us that we agreed with her decision.

The family was unanimous in its support. "She asked each of us when we talked to her from time to time, if we agreed with it," Xandra recalled.

"The first of September is the end, and I want to know that it is okay with you." And all of us said, "Yes, Mum, it's okay with us. No pain anymore. You can do whatever you want." She was a very good mother for us, and it was just terrible to see her in so much pain, with so much suffering. We would miss her, but we would manage.

I think it takes more courage to shorten your life than it does to live to the end, even with suffering. We all want to live a little longer if possible. But for her it was not possible. She knew that she was leaving us and she knew that we were grown up. It was very important for her to know that it was okay with us for her to leave us. We were very proud of her, that she could make the decision herself and not feel held back by her children.

"We could see that it was really the end," Dick said.

She could not go much further and she didn't want to. In those last two weeks she made all the arrangements that she wanted to make. We discussed whether she would have medicine that she could take herself or to have the doctor give her an injection. She knew exactly what she wanted and that was to have a doctor directly help her die. And that was a good choice. Her doctors felt the same way.

She did not like what morphine did to her mind, and at the end she insisted on having it stopped altogether so that she would be perfectly clear in what she said to us and what she understood us to say to her. At the end, she was wide awake and she laughed and made us all feel a little better. Her eyes were very bright and she talked very well. She seemed to be happy and she wanted us to be happy, too. We have good memories of our last moments together. Her life was so bad at the end that you could not question her decision. She asked all of us, and even her doctors, "Why should I go on for a longer time when there is no way back?" She understood that the end was near and that she could go now.

The actual decision was made forty days before the end, and the weeks got shorter and shorter. She wanted to have complete control. She organized her own cremation and funeral and the flowers and the letters. She did everything herself in advance. She planned her own death and even beyond it. At the very end she could do nothing, but she had expected that and had made her preparations days and even weeks before. The process of dying is not at the moment of death. It begins long before that. We lost her a little bit at a time, long before she actually died. That made the events at the end not so terrible.

She finally asked, "How long now? Another whole day? Why so long?" She was very sick then. She could change the forty days up to the last minute—put it off or move it up. It was just an arbitrary figure. She had pushed the date back herself several times because she thought she was doing okay. But she also knew when she had had enough. By that time she took so much morphine that she could not always recognize us, and she hated feeling helpless. She was very ill, and if she had not done this she probably would not have lived more than another few days.

On that last day, nature stepped in. She had a lot of trouble breathing or talking and was very sick. She decided on her own to move the date up one whole day to the thirty-first of August. She had a lot of water in her lungs, and it became an emergency quite quickly. The doctor gave her medication to get rid of the water through her kidneys. It did help dry her out, and in two hours she was breathing better, but she was so frightened by having trouble breathing that she decided she did not want to have to go through it any more. She said "That was enough. Do the euthanasia now, not tomorrow."

The doctor had come in the morning and discussed it with her. However, in the afternoon, when she became very ill, the doctor came to see her again. She was quite panicked and afraid that she would not even make it through the night. She wanted to have her death under her own control. She did not want to die by chance sometime in the middle of the night. The doctors were quite prepared and could arrange to do everything that same evening. This was all understood in advance. Most of the arrangements had been made about three weeks before, including an examination by another doctor to get a second opinion.

We were all here when she died. Also, her sister came, and my daughter's boyfriend. He knew her well and he wanted to be here to be of help. We spent the whole evening with her. We could say everything we wanted. There was plenty of time to go upstairs during the evening. We went one by one and we went together, some of us four or five times. We were under no pressure. It was already almost midnight and the doctor said if we wanted to talk to her, even until two or three o'clock, it would be no problem. We said "I love you" and "You are a wonderful mother," and there was really nothing else to say. There were no afterthoughts: "Oh I should have talked about this" or "I should have said that." We had said everything many times.

The four of us sat on her bed. Her choice was very simple, one injection with a sedative to make her very deeply asleep, and the second with curare to stop the breathing. The children were in the room for the first injection. Before that we said good-bye, and then I stayed alone and held her for the rest of the time while she got the second injection. It was very quick and very humane. We all felt that it was good that she did it this way. It was immediately evident. We never asked why or why not; we had no doubts about the whole situation.

After the death Dutch law requires that a coroner be called, only the coroner, not the police. On the telephone he asks if this was a natural death. As soon as the doctor says that it was not a natural death, the coroner has to come. This was not very pleasant. Everyone must leave the room, the door is closed and nothing can be touched until the coroner arrives. The needle must still be in the arm. The coroner must make a decision about whether this is acceptable euthanasia or a crime, even though all the arrangements had been made and the papers signed weeks before. He already knew that she was dying of cancer and planned to have euthanasia. We were all waiting downstairs and the coroner went up to look at everything. He must make a decision right away, while the doctor is there. After the coroner says it's okay, you can call for someone to remove the body. This was all very unpleasant, but it is still the law. Eventually the law may change further so that this step will not be necessary. That would be utopia.

Before this we did not know any family that had had euthanasia. Now that we have been through this experience, other families have talked to us about it many times. We also think that she chose the right moment. She was in so much pain and she was so frightened of what her illness was doing to her. We have had no second thoughts and no regrets. We were glad that we could support her.

The Netherlands, a Social Laboratory

In the 1970s the Netherlands became the first modern country to legalize physician-assisted dying. In so doing it initiated a social experiment that is being watched by much of the world and will probably be adopted in some form in the United States. Critics of the Dutch experience—and there are many—disapprove of this approach to suffering at the end of life, are appalled by the popularity that it has gained so rapidly in Holland, and do not want to see any aspect of it imported here. But the needs of those who must face painful deaths are the same in both cultures, and the Dutch experience, imperfect though it may be, deserves close analysis. It is as important to acknowledge the benefits of assisted dying as it is to recognize the risks that should be avoided.

The movement to legalize physician-assisted dying in the Netherlands began in 1973 with the Leeuwarden case, in which a family doctor was prosecuted for giving a lethal injection of morphine to her mother, who lived in a nursing home.[2] The mother was seventy-eight years old and in severe pain. She had repeatedly asked her daughter to help her die. The daughter finally acquiesced and was promptly charged with manslaughter. A great deal of public sympathy arose for the daughter. After two years the court found her guilty under existing law but sentenced her to only one week in prison and then suspended even that sentence. This tolerant stance by the court triggered a legal debate on the justification for any laws against physician-assisted dying under similar circumstances, a debate that continues today. It extended to religious groups, the medical community, ethicists, and much of the general public.

THE SOCIAL, LEGAL, AND ECONOMIC CLIMATE

Holland is a small country with a population of about fifteen million. It is racially and culturally homogeneous compared with the United States. Abject poverty and homelessness are rare, and the gap between rich and poor is relatively narrow. It enjoys a long tradition of tolerance. Jewish communities in cities like Amsterdam thrived for centuries until they were demolished by the Nazis. Even under the stress of their own suffering, many Dutch families took great risks hiding their Jewish neighbors. More recently, comprehensive sexual education in the schools and wide availability of sexual information have been credited with reducing Holland's levels of teenage pregnancy and abortion to the lowest in the Western world, even though abortion is available on request there. Similarly, progressive attitudes toward drug abuse have brought easy access to both drugs and treatment, resulting in low levels of addiction. Public moralizing and criticism are not common. The Dutch philosophy is more concerned with living one's own life well than in overseeing the lives of others. In this environment the seeds of physician-assisted dying fell on fertile soil.

The controversy over assisted dying came up at a time when Dutch cultural life was already undergoing significant change.[3] The trend of Dutch thinking in the 1960s and 1970s was toward increasing levels of autonomy and self-determination. Resolution of the abortion issue solidified the rights of women. Authority was challenged and established practices questioned in an atmosphere of social change. As the value of the individual increased, a comprehensive welfare state was created. The churches were carried along with this reform. Traditional thinking was bent to meet the needs of a less submissive and more secularized society. Holland, with its long tradition of religious tolerance, is now home to about fifty different religions. The major Protestant churches, primarily the Reformed and the Dutch Reformed, debated and eventually supported assisted dying. The Dutch Roman Catholic Church, one of the most progressive, has accepted use of oral contraceptives as a personal decision, but strongly opposes assisted dying.

There is other opposition to assisted dying in Holland. About one thousand physicians have collectively spoken out strongly against it. Conservative religious groups continue to voice their opposition. The Christian Democratic Party, central in the coalition government, opposes physician-assisted dying and has successfully blocked legalization that would provide physician immunity. Nonetheless, assisted dying has gained wide public support, and most opponents are now resigned to its success.

Because a physician is invariably and often openly involved in assisted dying, it is widely assumed that the movement began with the medical profession. In fact, physician-assisted dying in Holland arose from public debate and demand and from decisions by the courts, beginning with the Leeuwarden case. It was eventually accepted by a relatively conservative medical profession.[4]

The relation of the legal system to the medical profession is entirely different in Holland than in the United States. The large number of lawsuits against doctors in this country, and the huge settlements that often ensue, have created an entire "legal-protective" industry, with attorneys who specialize in medical cases, and insurance requirements that add significantly to the cost of medical care. American physicians have been forced to practice "defensive" medicine, relying on far more tests and documentation than are medically necessary. The Dutch physician is not similarly burdened. Malpractice is a medical concern rather than a legal one, to be judged by the medical community, not in court. Holland is not a litigious society, and few suits are brought against doctors. It is widely felt that they do the best they can, and they continue to enjoy a high level of trust and respect. As physician-assisted dying has gained acceptance in Holland, there is no evidence of loss of trust in the medical profession. Indeed, many commentators claim that the reputation of the profession has gained by taking on this new responsibility.

The Dutch legal system also differs significantly from our own, in that it allows some practices to be "legally tolerated" even though they are technically unlawful. The tendency in Holland is to allow a social issue to evolve by tolerating it but not legalizing it until it has a chance to mature and be thoroughly tested. The way that cases of assisted dying are handled in Holland is a good example.[5] According to the law, anyone who euthanizes another person, even at his request, will be punished by imprisonment for up to twelve years. A lesser penalty is assigned to a physician assisting in suicide. To avoid these penalties, the physician is required to notify a special prosecutor after she has helped a patient to die. If the coroner agrees that the patient did indeed have an appropriate illness and that the guidelines were met, he notifies the prosecutor that he sees no evidence of wrongdoing. The prosecutor then usually decides to excuse the case, even though it is "against the law." There is now considerable pressure in Holland to erase the legal ambiguity of assisted death by fully legalizing it.

It is unlikely that such a vague system of legal protection would ever be adopted in the United States. American physicians constantly work under the threat of malpractice suits and would demand strict, clear guidelines and immunity from prosecution before openly assisting people to die. We already have a de facto legal acceptance and protection, albeit at a later stage in prosecution. Several physicians have been prosecuted for assisting in patients' deaths, but none has yet been successfully convicted of a crime if the circumstances seemed appropriate. Timothy Quill's case was dismissed by a grand jury in New York State, and Jack Kevorkian underwent three trials, all of which failed to convict him or to prevent him from participating in more deaths, now numbering more than one hundred. Compassion is a strong motivation, and physicians are increasingly willing to break restrictive laws in order to provide relief for their patients.

Economic approaches to illness and death also divide the two countries. Health care financing remains a critical issue in the United States, but Holland has evolved a national system that includes public and private insurance. The coverage is extensive and applies to virtually all residents. The medical community has developed a few restrictions, such as age limitations for organ transplantation. Whatever reasons patients and families in Holland may have for requesting physician-assisted dying, they are never based on fear of financial loss or ruin. Total care is provided for as long as one lives. Health care in the United States falls far short of this ideal, and, as we have seen, financial concerns contribute to the demand for physician-assisted death.

PHYSICIAN AND PATIENT

Dutch citizens enjoy a long-term personal relationship with at least one physician, their family doctor or *huisarts*.[6] Each of these physi-

cians cares for about 2,300 individuals, often in a single neighbor-
hood. Theirs is an office and house-call practice, allowing them to
know entire families well. They are paid for the number of patients
they serve, not on a fee-for-service basis. It is the family doctor whom
a patient usually turns to with a request for physician-assisted dying.
The physician is well qualified to evaluate not only the patient's
medical and psychological condition but also the level of family support or evidence of family pressure. In general, the physician-patient
relationship is close. Dutch physicians who assist in dying consider
it to be a moral and professional responsibility. Because most prefer
to be present at the time of death, more than 80 percent of the assisted deaths are brought on by drugs administered by the physician—that is, euthanasia rather than assisted suicide.

The United States practices far more institutionalized medicine. Eighty percent of our deaths take place in hospitals or nursing
homes. Many families now prefer that death not take place at home.
In Holland about half of all deaths are at home, where family, physician, and clergy can all be present. Assisted dying, its notoriety
notwithstanding, is relatively rare; the vast majority of deaths at
home are from the underlying diseases, with the patient receiving
the best care that a supportive health system can provide. Critics of
physician-assisted dying in Holland focus on the fact that the Dutch
have not developed a hospice program as an alternative. But a family doctor who lives nearby and can come to the patient's home once
or even several times a day has many advantages over our home hospice program. Very few medical deaths in the United States take
place in hospice institutions, and it is widely acknowledged that
many of these people would prefer to die at home if they had a
choice.

Our high degree of specialization has been at the expense of
family doctors, who now attend only a small percentage of our families. However, I do not think that this picture is as totally different
as it seems to be for the patient who wishes to have help in dying.
Many internists fill the role of family physician and know their pa-

tients well and over long periods of time. Most people who are seriously ill and near death from chronic diseases, be it cancer or AIDS or respiratory failure, have at least one physician, perhaps a specialist, who has known the patient for years. The physician has watched the illness progress, and she has seen the patient's reaction to it. She probably has not been in the patient's home, but she has had an opportunity to get to know those family members who are the immediate care givers. In the American health care system, this physician is the logical person for the patient to turn to with his concerns about how and when he will die. With a little effort she can evaluate the depth and reasons for the patient's request and the position of at least some of the family, including their ability to care for the patient at home. Our inability to reproduce the family doctor relationships of Holland is not in itself a reason why we cannot provide physician assisted dying in a responsible fashion.

THE GUIDELINES

Dutch physicians and courts have developed a set of rules to be applied to assisted dying, rules that are more like guidelines than legal requirements.[7] Both criticized and praised, these guidelines have been incorporated in most proposals for legislation in the United States.

a. The request must be voluntary and must come from a competent patient.
b. It must be a durable, firm request, repeated several times over a period of weeks.
c. The patient must be fully informed about the decision and able to understand and evaluate the options.
d. The patient must be experiencing intolerable and hopeless suffering (either physical or mental).[8]
e. All alternatives must have been tried or rejected by the patient.
f. A second physician must see and evaluate the patient.
g. The nature of the death must be recorded on the death certificate and reported to the public prosecutor's office.

Evaluating the Dutch Experience

Writers outside of Holland, on both sides of the issue of physician-assisted dying, have cited the Dutch experience, usually to support their already established viewpoints. These arguments generally exclude conservative religious concerns, which are essentially the same in both countries. Authors who endorse physician-assisted dying, including Margaret Battin, Helga Kuhse, Sidney Wanzer, and Timothy Quill, suggest that the Dutch system is a noteworthy experiment, if not a model for what should take place in the United States.[9] They feel that the guidelines established are adequate, or nearly so. It should be noted that these same guidelines were adopted, essentially intact, in drafting the state proposals in Washington, California, and Oregon. Opponents, including Carlos Gomez, Alexander Capron, and Herbert Hendin, feel that the guidelines and safeguards in Holland are inadequate and often ignored, and that the program there is proof of the danger of a "slippery slope" hazarded by liberalization of the law governing physician-assisted dying.[10]

One of the major areas of intentional misunderstanding is the number of physician-assisted deaths that take place in the Netherlands each year. The data are limited, but some of the exaggerations are not. Two internal studies have provided most of the available information: the Remmelink report and an article by Gerrit van der Wal and colleagues.[11] Their findings were similar: euthanasia accounted for about 2,300 deaths in 1991–92. A much smaller number, 400 deaths, were physician-assisted suicides. The total of 2,700 voluntary deaths represents about 2 percent of all deaths that year. At this point the misunderstandings begin.

The study reported an additional 1,000 deaths in which assistance in dying was not specifically requested by the patient immediately beforehand. Most of these deaths involved people who had previously requested assisted dying but were later either unconscious or too bewildered by drugs or pain to update the request.[12] The common factor in most of these cases was extreme illness, suffering, and inability to communicate. The alleged incompetence of these patients to express their wishes to die placed them in a separate category, outside of the Dutch definition of voluntary euthanasia. The possibility obviously exists, though, that this group may have included some wrongful deaths. The inclusion of these patients as a separate figure in the Remmelink report has singled them out for special study and criticism and has called attention in Holland and elsewhere to the moral and legal problem that such patients present.

The Remmelink report also estimated that an additional 17 percent of all deaths were secondary to the use of narcotics to control pain (a practice that is widespread in the United States as well). Finally, another 18 percent of deaths were due to the discontinuation of or abstention from medical treatment, practices that are accepted and widely practiced here. Thus it was estimated that 35 percent of all deaths occurred under circumstances that are commonplace and legal in the United States and are not included in our definition of active euthanasia or assisted suicide. The study was thus misleading in its comprehensiveness, yielding a total of nearly 38 percent of all deaths in Holland that were grouped together under the heading "Medical Decisions Concerning the End of Life." This gave fuel to erroneous statements that a very large percentage of all deaths were physician assisted when the actual figure was no more that 3 percent, even if one includes those in which assistance was given although it was not specifically requested by the patient immediately beforehand. What is clear from both of these studies is the need for additional reliable data, preferably through better reporting.

The final note of concern about physician-assisted death in the Netherlands is the low rate of reporting. Although it has always been a criminal offense for the physician not to report such deaths, almost half of them still go unreported.[13] Steps are now being taken to understand the problem and to correct it. The reasons given for not reporting include the burden of legal review on the physician, the intrusion of legal review on the family, and the feeling that physician-assisted dying is a private concern of the patient and physician that should not involve the law.[14] Obviously any assisted death that falls even marginally outside of the legally accepted guidelines is unlikely to be reported. One of the solutions being considered is to transfer responsibility for overseeing physician-assisted dying to the medical profession itself, possibly the Royal Dutch Medical Society, or to some appointed body, using notification and evaluation procedures that do not involve the law. In cases of flagrant abuse of the guidelines or of suspected wrongful death, the courts would continue to be involved. The courts have treated nonreporting as a minor infraction if the major guidelines have been followed.

Much attention has been given to Dutch physician-assisted dying by critics in other countries. The Dutch have created a model that many admire but one that is clearly flawed. Closer at hand, in the Netherlands itself, the movement has found a high level of public support. Forty percent of the population favored euthanasia in 1966. By 1975, during discussion of the Leeuwarden case, the figure had risen to 52 percent, and in 1986 it was 67 percent.[15] These figures correspond closely to similar evaluations of public support in the United States. But the Dutch are wholesome, fun-loving people who enjoy a high standard of living in a socially advanced country. They are certainly not preoccupied with death and dying, nor are they plagued by concerns about Nazi-like excesses, though they experienced them firsthand. They see themselves as having addressed a very human problem—intense and hopeless suffering at the end of life—in a very humane fashion. Moreover, they consider it their solution to meet the needs of their own society; they do not consider it necessarily a product for export. If outsiders wish to look in and see what is happening, the doors stand wide. The Dutch experiment is being watched closely—by some out of fear that its success may spread, and by others in hope that its success will spread.

It is entirely wrong to expect members of one profession as a regular matter of course to jeopardize their whole careers in order to save the rest of us the labor and embarrassment of changing the law.
Antony Flew

5 Physicians' Concerns

The blossoming of modern medicine began in the 1930s and 1940s with the development of drugs that could actually cure disease. The physician, who up to this time could usually do little more than make a reasonably accurate diagnosis and then wait with the patient while nature took its course, was transformed into a true healer. It is hard now even for physicians to appreciate what a major step this was, or how very recent. Research thrived and curative surgery was extended to every part of the body. Remarkably, this rate of growth and development has not yet even begun to slow down. It is no wonder that we marvel at what can be done to treat disease or that the new focus is on treatment and more treatment.

Everyone should be happy, physician, patient, and society alike—but they are not. All too often the modern physician is seen as a scientist and technician first and only incidentally, if at all, as a caring and compassionate person. A plethora of tests and procedures can leave little time for explanations and support. Modern physicians have been pulled away from the traditional bedside by the power of new medicines that demand most of their time and intellect but provide results beyond the imagination of their forebears. It is ironic that the doctor who can now treat patients so effectively has lost much of the personal touch. Holding a patient's hand was once commonplace and essential, if for no other reason than there was little else that could be done. Indeed, the laying on of hands was an ancient form of healing. Now some physicians find personal contact an embarrassment. Why try to comfort patients when you could be treating them?

The burgeoning complexity of modern medicine has required a high degree of specialization, with a corresponding loss of interest and knowledge about other equally specialized areas. Sophisticated tools require extensive use of the hospital. This centralization of equipment and expertise has lead to the demise of the house call and to less intimate understanding of patient and family together. In every advanced disease there comes a time when further treatment is futile and a person's care and comfort may be provided better at home. As a society we have sometimes forgotten this wisdom, assuming instead that more can be done in the hospital.

We have recently begun to witness a loss of confidence in the medical profession and in physicians as individuals. There has been a move away from trusting that the physician could do no wrong to requiring a second opinion to be sure that she is right. Now, just as she is mastering the new science at her disposal, the doctor is under pressure to be a better physician, to be more compassionate and caring, to show more concern for patients as people and not just as diseases to be treated.

Against this background of change, the physician is being asked secretly—and in the future, perhaps, more openly—to help her most troubled patients end their suffering a little sooner. In confronting such a request the physician must deal with her personal and professional reservations as well as conflicting moral values. As members of the general population, physicians share various backgrounds with respect to religion, family, parents and parenting, friendships, goals, love of life, enjoyment of leisure, and other values. Added to these is an extensive and elite education and membership in a very respected but demanding profession.

The physician is vested with real authority, from her contractual relationship with the patient, unwritten but clearly understood. The privilege of access to the bodies, minds, and sufferings of other people is given in exchange for providing treatment and care. Licensing by the state confers an element of legal authority, almost like that of a public officeholder. At the same time, though the dynamic of the relationship has changed, the physician continues to exercise personal influence over the patient, who in extreme cases endows the physician with Godlike qualities. Some patients like to confer this honor on physicians, and many physicians enjoy the role.

Medicine and religion were closely related in antiquity and were one and the same through more than a millennium of early Christianity. Today this superhuman role owes its existence to the capacity of the modern physician to cure disease and prolong life. The converse, however, is not generally accepted—that the physician can openly do anything to shorten life, regardless of the circumstances. The result is that playing God with human lives has become a one-way street: extending life is expected, shortening life is illegal. James Rachels pointed out this inconsistency in paraphrasing a statement made by David Hume more than two hundred years ago. "If it is for God alone to decide when we shall live and when we shall die, then we 'play God' just as much when we cure people as when we kill them. We alter the length of a person's life when we save it just as much as when we take it."[1]

This chapter examines the personal, professional, and ethical concerns that are raised for physicians by issues as profound as assisted dying. In it I shall provide a representative physician's point of view in hopes of helping the reader to understand some of the problems that assisted dying presents to doctors. The discussion may also help physicians to better formulate their own views and understand the views of their colleagues.

Personal Concerns

Man is the only animal that can contemplate its own mortality. The price we pay for understanding the value of life is fear of death. Personal attitudes toward death inevitably influence the behavior of physicians. It has been suggested that doctors fear death even more than the general population does and that this fear may send some into the profession in the first place.[2] Certainly young people entering medical school bring with them the same experiences as others, including deaths in their immediate families. Although our attitudes toward death are deeply ingrained in our psyches, they are also a function of exposure and experience, both of which can be avoided or confronted as one wishes. Many physicians learn to deal effectively with dying patients and their families. Uncomfortable at first, they may find it easier with time. In the process, the physician has an opportunity to work through her own fear of death and begin to see it as a natural process.

One of the patients who taught me the most about coping with death was the widow of a minister from Virginia. She had been treated for years at the National Cancer Institute for leiomyosarcoma, a rare smooth-muscle tumor that had formed in the wall of the vena cava, a vein that carries blood to the heart. She had had several operations for the condition but finally moved to Minneapolis to live with her daughter when it became clear that her treatment options had been used up. At this point, I took over her care. She underwent a few new chemotherapy regimens, none of which did much good. The tumor was progressing slowly, and she preferred just to be kept comfortable. One evening I stopped off to see her when she was in the hospital, and she confronted me with some alarming questions. What is it like to die? Why does it take so long to die? What happens when we die? How do we die? What happens after we die? Although I was about forty years old at the time, the questions were too direct and the subject matter too sensitive for me to deal with. I literally fled.

At that time a psychologist, John Brantner, was on the faculty of the University of Minnesota. I had heard him speak on death and dying, and I asked him whether he would like to interview my patient for his own interest, suggesting that perhaps he might at the same time be of some help to her. He visited her, and a few days later he asked me whether I had spoken to her at all. I admitted that I had not. "It would be a good experience for you," he said. "Sit down with her when you have plenty of time and just let her talk. She doesn't expect you to have answers to all those questions. She is just frustrated and a little frightened and wants someone to talk to. You will be doing yourself a real favor if you do it." That Saturday afternoon, I pulled up a chair beside her bed. Our talk took two hours and quite a few Kleenexes. I do not think that there is any aspect of death or dying, be it personal, medical, or religious, that we did not cover. Without a doubt, she was the teacher and I the student. I grew up a lot in one afternoon.

After my patient left the hospital, I went to see her once a week at her daughter's home, not far from where I lived. I can still count on the fingers of two hands the number of patients for whom I have made home visits. Our conversation went on from where we left off in the hospital. Sometimes her daughter would join us. I was amazed at how much my visits seemed to help them both, even though medically they accomplished nothing at all. Eventually my patient died, peacefully and comfortably. I continued to exchange Christmas cards with her family for many years.

By their behavior, physicians display a wide range of attitudes toward the death of their patients. Some deal well with dying patients, staying at hand throughout the process and providing support. Others avoid dying patients as much as they can, particularly as the end draws near. They find excuses to be elsewhere and turn as much of the personal contact as possible over to other people—

colleagues, subordinates, and particularly nurses. These physicians may make themselves available before or after the time of death, but they are too uncomfortable to share the actual event with dying patients and grieving families. This avoidance extends beyond death. Rarely do any physicians send letters of condolence or attend a funeral or memorial service for a patient.

Another way that physicians can avoid confronting death is by distancing themselves intellectually from the dying process. This is done by shifting the responsibility from physician to disease. Discontinuing a respirator, for example, is letting the patient die of his underlying disease; giving high doses of morphine is relieving pain, even though respiration is knowingly suppressed. Both of these strategies lessen the physician's feelings of having any direct responsibility for death.

DEATH AS FAILURE

Closely related to fear of death is the concept of death as a form of failure. With the emphasis in the medical profession on successful treatment, many physicians look on the death of a patient as a personal shortcoming. At one time, death was accepted and respected, even by doctors. Now death is the enemy, and the battleground is the hospital. When a sick patient enters the hospital, he is taking a significant step toward confronting his own mortality. At a conscious level he realizes that the hospital is where you go to get better and that the opposite of this is to get worse and even to die. Unlike a century ago, the hospital is now where the healing hands really are. The physician feels this responsibility, too, and often she succeeds in treating the illness. When she fails, though, she may feel guilty because she could not or did not do more. In a sense it is indeed failure: the best that medicine could offer did not cure the disease or at least prolong life. It is important to distinguish, though, between failure and fault. Many patients with cancer eventually die of their disease. But there is no fault and there should be no guilt on the part of people who did their best.

Doctors sometimes find it difficult to maintain the same relationship with a patient for whom treatment no longer helps. They are trained to restore health, and when this isn't possible, they often unconsciously pull back from the patient. The common goal of working together to beat the disease is abandoned, and the patient can usually sense it. A medical oncologist observed, "When we make rounds on the oncology floor, we initially go into the room and do all we can. But when there is 'nothing left to do,' we don't go in anymore. We stop outside the door and talk in hushed voices. The general excuse is something like, 'Well, we're not doing anything,' or 'The family wants privacy.' But that's not true. If they didn't want us to come in, they would tell us. But that is not what you hear. They feel abandoned. It's noticed and it's not good."

The sense of frustration and even failure can be projected onto the patient. As a surgeon who does heart transplants expressed it: "Occasionally patients become discouraged after transplantation and decide to discontinue their immunosuppression. At times like that I feel betrayed by the patient and even angry. The patient had opted for the full power of modern medical technology, and we commit a tremendous effort to making it work. More important, we selected him and allocated a scarce resource, the heart or lung or whatever is being transplanted, an organ that could have been given to someone else. If the patient then decides, because of some quality-of-life issue, to stop taking their drugs and die, I feel that the whole system has been let down."

THE PAINFUL TRUTH

Physicians are often uncomfortable discussing goals and options with patients when both are clearly limited. Until recently, it was considered an unnecessary infliction of pain even to mention the possibility of eventual death, and the topic is still routinely avoided in many countries and cultures.[3] Some patients really would prefer not to know what may lie ahead, and no sensitive physician would force unwanted information on such a person. These people, though, identify themselves in unmistakable terms: "I don't really want a long discussion about it. Please just do whatever you think is best and take care of things."

But a physician's fear of open discussion can compromise the patient's right to know the truth about the chances of success for various treatment options. Few physicians will volunteer the information that a disease will eventually be fatal and offer to review the predictable course of the illness and the possible variations that might be expected. Even when patients bring up end-of-life issues, many physicians avoid discussing them. They feel that they are obligated to hold out hope, even when they know there is none. They see a narrow line between hope and reality, and they prefer to tread on the side of hope, regardless of the wishes of the patient. Some physicians even deceive themselves by offering additional treatment to foster unrealistic hope.

Such physicians may use a variety of offhand and sometimes glib ways of dismissing hard questions—answering, for example, "If you tell me how long I am going to live, I'll tell you how long you are going to live." The question of when I am going to die is not an easy one to ask. It takes courage and forethought even to bring it up, and it deserves a reasoned answer, including the likely minimum and maximum of remaining life and a description of the vagaries of the disease itself. Only with accurate information can people intelligently select their treatment options, options that may be very straightforward at the beginning but exceedingly difficult later when the disease is advanced and death is approaching. Knowing the truth helps the patient explore the short- and long-term possibilities and even to think about the end earlier in the course of the disease, when he is relatively well and psychologically able to deal with the issues involved. Later, when remote possibilities of dying have become imminent, the opportunity may have been lost.

The outgrowth of patient autonomy is that physicians must be prepared to answer questions and engage in fruitful discussion, all the while being sensitive to clues from the patient and providing their own clues about their willingness to confront and discuss difficult issues. Indeed, the physician may have a legal as well as a moral obligation to provide the patient with important information. Two physicians in California failed to discuss a poor prognosis with a patient who had cancer of the pancreas, even after it recurred. They lost a suit brought by the patient's family.[4] In an editorial in the *New England Journal of Medicine,* Marcia Angell commented on the "tendency of physicians to rely on nonverbal communication and patient initiatives in exchanging information," rather than directly and openly establishing the patient's wishes.[5] Some physicians receive far more hints or even requests concerning assisted dying than do others; they must somehow seem more open to discussion of the subject, or at least make it clear that they will not be affronted by it.

Until recently, it was easier for the physician to deal with an adverse diagnosis or end-of-life questions because she had to do it only with the family. A strong moral and legal tradition demanded that some close relative should know—but not the patient. Even now there is a tendency for physicians to discuss sensitive medical issues with the families of competent patients rather than with the patients themselves, a practice that undermines the patient's autonomy and isolates him from both family and his physician.[6]

A surgeon I knew at the University of Minnesota Hospital had a patient who had been transferred from elsewhere in the state following surgery for cancer of the large bowel. The patient's problem was continuing bowel obstruction and a fistula, from which liquid stool was discharging through his partially healed surgical wound onto his abdominal wall. The surgeon, a senior member of the department, performed two or three operations to try to close these fistulas and reestablish continuity of his intestinal tract. Each of these failed. There is an adage in medicine that when you keep doing the right thing but it fails, think of cancer. This was in the mind of all the medical staff, but there was no evidence that this man had any residual tumor from his original operation.

The man's wife, a schoolteacher like her husband, had taken a leave of absence from her job to be with him. Their home was two hundred miles away, so she arranged for her parents to take care of their children and got a room near the hospital. She spent many hours, day and night, at her husband's bedside.

Finally, after his last operation, the pathology report showed that a recurrence of his tumor was indeed causing the continuing obstruction and the fistula. His wife was appalled by this news and insisted that her husband not be told. The staff acceded to her wishes. Moreover, the surgeon who had operated on him and was primarily responsible for him began to avoid him altogether, unprepared as he was to sit down and discuss the problem openly.

But the patient was perceptive. He noticed a change in the attitudes of the doctors and nurses taking care of him that made him suspect that they were withholding information. He began to be more aggressive with his questioning, particularly of the nurses who were alone with him at night. Their discomfort finally brought the situation to the attention of the hospital's ethics committee, which is charged with helping to resolve conflicts between patients, families, and the medical staff. It was clear to the committee that the patient had every right to know about his condition and that everyone except his wife wanted him to know. The committee decided that the primary responsibility of the hospital and the doctors was to the patient and not to the wife, that it was wrong for the senior surgeon to withhold the information, and that the patient's questions should be answered truthfully and directly.

To try to avoid unnecessary confrontation we notified the wife and told her that we were going to talk to her husband the next day, explaining his condition and answering his questions as well as we could. After a long silence she said, "Oh no, you are not. I am going to tell him tonight. It's my responsibility. I created the problem and I will solve it." And she did. They had a long conversation late at night in which she explained what we had told her in detail. She had enough information to answer most of his questions. She must have done it very well, for the next day he was cheerful and happy and loving again with his wife and grateful to the doctors and nurses who were taking care of him. He never left the hospital but died there about two weeks later, at peace with himself and with his family.

FEARSOME RESPONSIBILITY

Most human beings share a repugnance for causing death. War has its own rules, the essence of which is "kill or be killed," and some see capital punishment as fair retribution for heinous crimes. These exceptions prevail because the conditions on which they depend are relatively impersonal and can be rationalized. But there is nothing impersonal about discontinuing an intravenous medication that supports blood pressure and heart action, about "pulling the plug" of a respirator, or about giving a drug that stops respiration. The relation of the action to the ensuing death is direct, obvious, and devastating. It should not be otherwise. Although two of these activities are accepted both in principle and in practice, the ability of individual physicians to participate varies a great deal from one to another. As we have seen, many physicians insist upon the subtle difference between withdrawing treatment to allow a person to die and more actively helping a person to die. The responsibility that a physician is willing to take with a dying patient is a very personal decision, and no one should be forced to help another person die. Some doctors and lawmakers are also concerned that legal permission to assist in a person's death could become a legal obligation. This possibility seems remote indeed. This has not been the case for individual physicians in removing life support or performing abortions, both of which have become widely accepted, so there is no reason why it should be different in physician-assisted dying. What is accepted in principle need not be accepted in practice by the individual doctor.[7]

Some observers fear that participation in assisted dying would desensitize physicians to the value of life. My own experience, and that of all physicians whom I have spoken to, is just the opposite. The value of life assumes a new dimension when you have personally helped to bring it to an end.

I was a resident at the Massachusetts General Hospital in Boston in 1965. This was before there were any formal ethics committees and the law of double effect was unknown to us. A twenty-five-year-old victim of an auto accident had suffered a serious head injury. He was in a coma, on a respirator, in what would now be considered a persistent vegetative state, and remained so, without change, for many weeks. Members of his family came to see him every day and tentatively asked whether there had been any improvement. There never was. The neurologist explained to them that the severity of the brain injury left no chance of recovery. Finally the family began to ask how long the patient might stay in this state and to give other clues that the situation was exhausting them. As the weeks went by, visits from the family became less frequent and then stopped altogether.

We decided to hold a conference to discuss turning off the respirator. The family preferred not to attend but made it clear, through the father, that they did not want their son to live this way any longer. This ad hoc ethics committee was the first such conference held at that hospital. It was attended by a member of the hospital administration, the supervisor of the nursing service, several nurses caring for the patient, several physicians, a Catholic priest, a rabbi, a Protestant chaplain, and an attorney for the hospital. The nurses pointed out how demoralizing it was to take care of a beautiful young person for such a long time when there was clearly no hope for recovery. The hospital administrator said that ordinarily a person like this would be transferred to a nursing home or an extended care facility but that no such institutions would take a person on a respirator. He also pointed out that the hospital could not sustain the expense of the care indefinitely. The physicians involved with the young man's care remarked on the hopeless outlook and the fact that the family had stopped visiting and had requested that the supportive care be stopped. The minister and the rabbi said that the patient's life was over for himself, his family, and for God, and that it was all right for him to die. The priest surprised some of us by agreeing, changing the words to "useful life." The attorney pointed out that there was no legal precedent for or against removing life support, but he was aware that it was done from time to time. He felt that if everyone agreed, particularly the family, then the legal risks were acceptable.

The decision was made to turn off the respirator. The family was notified and came in together to see their loved one for one last time. The father wanted to be present when the respirator was turned off. Then the question was raised of who should actually do it. I was the chief resident and responsible for the service. Moreover, I had convened the conference, hoping at some level that this would be its recommendation. It gradually dawned on me that I was expected to take on the responsibility of turning off the machine. I did not like the idea at all and hoped that someone else would step forward. No one did. The issue was in my mind constantly for the next few days, as I sought the courage to make the final arrangements and set a date. Slowly, I began to feel that this might be a very important personal experience, to be dreaded but not to be avoided. Although uncomfortable and upsetting, it could be an opportunity to grow.

The time was set for Sunday morning. The father came with his own minister. Two nurses and another physician were also present. The minister said a short prayer. I disconnected the respirator and the patient died within a few minutes. His injury had left him totally paralyzed and unable to see or hear or feel any pain, so there was no significant reaction on his part. He made a few very shallow attempts at breathing and then stopped. We held hands together while the minister said another short prayer, and then we began to talk about the young man and what we had just done. His father thanked us for having explored the situation so thoroughly and for then having the courage to go through with it. The result of our introspection was that we had indeed actively taken the life of a human being, and that we had done the right thing.

BREAKING THE LAW

No physician who even considers helping a person die can overlook the fact that it is against the law in most states. It is also well known that there has never been a successful prosecution against a physician acting on the rational request of the patient or his family. The reasons for this are clear. If the circumstances are indeed appropriate, it would be difficult to find a prosecutor or a judge, not to mention a jury, that would not sympathize with the patient and wish that they too could have a compassionate physician if they were ever in similar circumstances.

Although prosecution may be rare, the threat is real. A few physicians have had to spend vast amounts of money to defend themselves. Although public opinion is usually in their favor, the publicity is not the sort that most practicing physicians seek. Finally, the threat of a medical malpractice suit is a serious and widely respected deterrent. Any member of a patient's family, however remote he or she might be from the patient in daily life, can accuse a physician of assisting in the death. More than any other single factor, including religion and personal ethics, the current illegality of physician-assisted dying is the single most cited deterrent among the physicians whom I interviewed.

It is clear, both legally and professionally, that doing less rather than more is safer for the physician. Physicians who help people die are extremely careful to make it appear to be a natural death or to be suicide. More often, the time-honored ethics of the profession, the personal discomfort involved, and the law all push the physician to maintain her distance by refusing even the most pathetic and needy patients who request help.

Legalization of physician-assisted dying would eliminate the threat of malpractice if the act met the required criteria. Physician, patient, family, the public, and law enforcement agencies would understand that if the legal requirements were observed, the physician could not be prosecuted. Passage of such laws would also help clarify several issues, including the definition of patient autonomy, the differences between passive and active euthanasia at practical and legal levels, and the responsibility of the physician to control suffering as opposed to prolonging life.

Professional Concerns

In addition to the physician's personal concerns about assisted dying, she must also take into consideration the concerns of medicine as a profession. Some of the rules of professional ethics and behavior are codified, while other, more general principles are tacitly understood. The professional societies that are the guardians of these rules are also responsible for updating them.

Personal integrity consists of having a stable set of values and principles that govern one's actions and words.[8] These values often include such general qualities as diligence, honesty, and reliability. Beyond personal integrity is the concept of professional integrity, which includes those elements and duties that identify a person as a physician. This more restrictive form of integrity is oriented around service to other people: professional competence, benefiting the patient, avoiding unnecessary harm, and justifying and maintaining the trust of the patient.

With issues as complex as assisted dying, elements of personal and professional integrity may come into conflict, particularly because the professional stance has traditionally opposed any such activity. To lessen this conflict would require broadening the definition of professional integrity. Leon Kass speaks firmly against this evolution, describing "medicine's outer limits," beyond which none may trespass: "This principle would establish strict outer boundaries—indeed, inviolable taboos—against those 'occupational hazards' to which each profession is especially prone. Within these outer limits, no fixed rules of conduct apply; instead, prudence—the wise judgment of the man-on-the-spot—finds and adopts the best course of action in the light of the circumstances. But the outer limits themselves are fixed, firm, and nonnegotiable."[9]

Others argue just the opposite, that concepts of professional integrity can indeed include assisted dying. This stance is based on the observation that traditional concepts have changed and are changing, that medicine has several goals, not just healing, that death is not necessarily a harm, that trust is unlimited in direction and scope, and that abandonment can include failure to relieve unwanted suffering.[10]

Yet another camp suggests that assisted suicide should not be a medical event at all but rather a community-social issue, thereby not requiring any move away from the traditional tenants of professional integrity.[11] We have already seen, however, that the medical profession is uniquely qualified and therefore expected to deal with assisted dying. The community and society will have their say through the laws they pass, but final responsibility for doing or not doing will rest with the physician. It is also clear that physicians' personal interests and concepts of integrity are changing and are pushing more and more strongly against the restrictions of the perceived integrity of the profession.

The professional ethic against physician-assisted dying dates to ancient Greece and the oath of Hippocrates. Until recently this oath was administered to all medical students as part of their graduation exercises. As a code of ethics, it dealt more with the concerns of the profession of medicine than with those of the patient. It has fallen short of the needs of modern medicine in so many respects that it has been all but dropped from our thinking. The oath was rarely mentioned by physicians interviewed in this study. Still, it remains one of the most quoted denunciations of physician-assisted dying. For this reason it deserves a closer look.

Although credited to Hippocrates, this document was almost certainly written by someone else, in the school of thought ascribed to Hippocrates, which lasted for about three hundred years after his death. Moreover, the conservative thinking expressed in the oath was probably that of one small group of physicians, the Pythagorean school, and not that of Hippocrates himself.[12] The oath has many proscriptions that are no longer observed. It prohibits surgery, "use of the knife—even on sufferers from bladder stone," when other writings attributed to Hippocrates acknowledged the need for such procedures. The oath also decries abortion. Finally, the oath declares that "I will neither give a deadly drug to anybody if asked for it nor will I make a suggestion to this effect." By most accounts this was written at a time when suicide was common and physicians frequently helped patients to die. It was only later, under the influence of Christianity, that censure of abortion and physician-assisted dying was solidified.

Medical Societies

Professional societies began in ancient times with the advent of the professions themselves and have continued to gain in influence to the present day. They set their members apart from the general public and identify and screen out unqualified practitioners. Regular meetings provide opportunities for education and for exchanges of ideas and information, as well as camaraderie among old friends and colleagues. At a public level, professional societies establish and maintain standards of practice. They oversee the quality of medical schools and evaluate and approve hospitals as centers for training in medical specialties. Finally, the state licensing board is an offshoot of the medical society, and its authorization is required in order to practice. Unquestionably, a major function of the medical society is to protect and further the interests of the society itself and of the group it represents.

The largest and most visible medical organization in the United States is the American Medical Association (AMA). The AMA supports one of the wealthiest and strongest political action committees in the country to further the interests of the medical profession as it perceives them. It is important to realize, however, that medical societies like the AMA and similar state organizations do not include or represent all members of the profession. Only about 40 percent of all practicing physicians in the United States belong to the AMA, and this number is dropping. Over the years, the AMA has been very conservative, fighting anything remotely resembling "socialized medicine." As a result of its conservative stance on many issues, it has lost the support of many liberal physicians. Although the AMA speaks for more physicians than any other organization in the United States and is looked upon by many as the voice of organized medicine, its views were so well known that its leadership was left out of most early discussions by the Clinton administration of possible health care reform that took place in 1993 and 1994.

The early history of the AMA is closely tied to the issue of abortion.[13] Because the parallels between assisted dying and abortion are numerous, this history is instructive. The AMA was founded in the 1850s to distinguish "regular" physicians, who had educations that prepared them for the practice of medicine, from "irregulars," who did not. An issue was needed to clarify this distinction, and abortion was suggested by Dr. Horatio Storer, an obstetrician from Boston. Regular physicians would not perform abortions. The nascent AMA seized upon this. Moreover, the members carried the issue to the legislatures of every state over the next few years, successfully criminalizing abortion at any time in pregnancy, except to save the life of the mother. After a final statement on abortion in 1871, the AMA lost interest in the issue for almost a century.

By the early 1960s about ten thousand abortions a year were being performed in U.S. hospitals. The American Law Institute recommended significant liberalization of the laws, and in the next few years, several states modified their statutes. Finally, in 1970, after three years of bitter debate between pro-life and pro-choice advocates, the AMA approved of abortion, essentially on demand. This decision took a heavy toll on membership. Nevertheless, I think that the AMA will someday reach a similar threshold over the issue of assisted dying, and there is every reason to believe that the sequence of events will be about the same. But it is such a divisive issue that the association would like to avoid it for as long as possible.

By defining the nature of professional duty as they see it, medical societies set rules of ethics and behavior for their members.[14] The AMA currently opposes physician-assisted dying on the grounds that the physician could no longer claim to be a pure healer, and the image of the profession would thus be damaged. In 1992 the judicial affairs council report of the AMA affirmed patient autonomy but stopped short of condoning any form of assisted dying, noting that "there is an autonomy interest in directing one's death, but this interest is more limited in the case of euthanasia than in the case of refusing life support."[15]

The problem with this reasoning is that the image of the medical profession is already tarnished precisely because of its self-centered and conservative attitudes toward many social issues. It is inconsistent to loudly proclaim support for patient autonomy but stop short of assisted dying, one of the most basic areas of autonomy. "The medical profession's repeated and firm rejection of any participation by physicians in assisted suicide begins to appear self-serving in its emphasis on a professional scrupulosity that seems blind to the expressed needs of the patients."[16]

Many physicians do not think that the image of the medical profession would be damaged by supporting assisted dying. A medical oncologist told me: "It probably would not make a difference. Patients really do want to know that their physicians are going to relieve their suffering, no matter what is involved." Another medical oncologist said, "It would enhance the image of medicine because patients would see it as addressing their real suffering, rather than abstract professional issues." And a neurologist declared: "It would soon be perceived as part of the physician's role in enabling people to die with dignity. That would not be a very big step for people to take."

A second but closely related objection by the AMA is concern about the effect of assisted dying on the physician-patient relation-ship. Not only would the image of the medical profession be tarnished, but so would that of the individual physicians. What patient would trust a physician who was known to have helped people die? If a patient were distressed enough to bring up the subject and the physician were to agree that the choice is a rational one and that assisted suicide is a reasonable alternative, would this not reinforce the patient's feelings of despair and worthlessness? Even a suggestion of agreement, the AMA speculated, might undermine any remaining hope.[17]

Open discussion with a physician would certainly confirm a person's suspicions that the situation was indeed desperate and life expectancy short—facts that would have to be confronted in any compassionate and meaningful conversation about how life would end. The possibility of assisted dying is too threatening to be brought up by a reticent or squeamish patient. Open discussion thus requires a physician who is also comfortable with at least talking about the subject. If the physician is to address the patient's concerns at all, she must acknowledge—and guard against—the risk that any sign of sympathy or agreement will be demoralizing. Beyond that, a reasoned and sympathetic evaluation of all of the alternatives should offset any fears that the physician is eager to help bring life to an end. The physician's responsibility is to, not for, the physician-patient relationship; cultivating that relationship protects the interests of both parties.[18]

I have seen very little evidence that approval of assisted dying would undermine patients' relationships with their physicians. Most patients interviewed in my study felt that knowledge that their physicians had helped others to die would either have no effect or would enhance their respect for their physicians. A cancer patient stated his position clearly: "My first criterion for a doctor is one who will give me the best chance to live a reasonable life for as long as possible. It would be a big added plus if the doctor would help me die if the end gets bad." I posed the same question to all of the physicians interviewed, and most felt it was not an issue. If the physician had a good reputation and was knowledgeable, conscientious and caring, they said, she would remain a fully qualified and highly desirable physician. A few patients with strong feelings against assisted dying would probably look elsewhere for their medical care, but most would not.

For an analogous situation I asked three gynecologists who occasionally do abortions whether they were ever questioned about the practice in principle by other patients. One had been, on a single occasion. When she replied that she did do abortions, the patient requested that her surgery (a hysterectomy) be done at a nearby Catholic hospital, but by the same gynecologist. Abortion seems at times to be a major public issue but a minor private one.

One colleague of mine who specializes in lung diseases had a patient leave his practice immediately after being told that the doctor would not consider aid in dying under the present legal restrictions. "She had been treated with radiation for Hodgkin's disease, and went on to develop severe radiation-induced lung disease," my colleague told me.

Over several years, she developed respiratory failure with complete loss of her former exercise capacity. She was very concerned that she would die a gasping and terribly painful death. She and her husband asked if I could provide a drug that she could have on hand to take when she felt that she had suffered enough. In principle, I had no problem with the idea of prescribing something and being of assistance in that sense. However, I am a practicing physician and provide health care delivery to a large number of people and did not want to risk compromising that and my future without serious thought. There was no question what the issue was from my point of view, and I was very open about it. I explained that I had a family to raise and that I had a lot of patients who depended on me, and that I could not legally do it. Our relationship was basically severed by my decision not to help. I could feel them pulling away from me over this. More to the point, if it had been legal, I would gladly have helped them.

The AMA currently holds that it is better to prohibit any form of assisted dying, for any reason whatsoever, than to face squarely the hard moral issue of responsibility to the dying patient who wants to die, or to grapple with the ethical nuances of assisted suicide versus euthanasia, degrees of suffering, and life expectancy. But the door to reasoned dissent may already be ajar. The 1992 judicial affairs council noted that "in certain, carefully defined circumstances, it would be humane to recognize that death is certain and suffering is great. However, the societal risks of involving physicians in medical interventions to cause patients' deaths is too great in this culture to condone euthanasia or physician assisted suicide at this time." Still, the council admitted, "a more careful examination of the issue is necessary."[19]

Medical Ethics and Moral Choices

Morality can be defined as our common understanding of what makes human conduct right or wrong.[20] Moral principles have evolved over the course of civilization, and they are still evolving. Being neither faultless nor perfect nor complete, morality is shaped by the needs and thinking of the times. As circumstances change, moral thought encounters conflicting values, where right and wrong are not clear, are subject to different interpretations, or are decided only slowly by an evolutionary process. Moral principles can also overlap and conflict with each other. This is the basis for the study of ethics.

Medicine has a formidable tradition of paternalism. "The doctor knows best" was not only repeated by generations of parents to their children, it was accepted quite blindly by the adults. Even now, a liver transplant surgeon described herself as her "patient's advocate" in urging the patient and family to let her attempt a second transplant after the first had failed. Unquestioning acceptance of physicians' recommendations has broken down significantly in the past fifty years. Explanations and consent are expected and often required. This transfer of power is still taking place, as patients and physicians seek a new balance point. Issues that challenge tradition, like assisted dying, fuel everyone's concerns as to who should be in charge.

The medical ethicist Edmund Pellegrino, M.D., feels that a high level of paternalism is demanded when the issue is assisted dying. He feels that physicians must determine whether patients are clinically depressed, are suffering unbearably, have resolved all psychological and spiritual problems, and can be classified as "extreme." Because physicians also control the availability and timing of assisted death, he feels that in such an interaction, patient autonomy is a fiction and the physician must retain control and make the final decision. He believes, furthermore, that the decision should never be in favor of assisted dying.[21] Pellegrino seems to view assisted dying as different from all other patient-physician interactions; elsewhere he gives patients far more credit, stating that "the best interests of the patient are intimately linked with their preferences, from which are derived our primary duties towards them."[22]

A widely accepted limitation on autonomy is that the private activity of one individual or group should not interfere with the rights or well-being of others. Daniel Callahan, former director of the Hastings Center, extends the concept of *others,* asserting that the physician's role in society turns her involvement with a patient's death into a social act rather than a private one, with implications for the entire community. For this reason, the enlistment of a physician's help opens the elected death of a person to social, moral, and legal considerations.[23] This argument attempts to globalize an intensely private matter by extending the physician's realm of responsibility. No precedent exists for such public supervision or control. The Supreme Court declared abortion to be a matter of privacy between a woman and her physician. Although physicians must report certain diseases, such as tuberculosis and syphilis, to public health authorities, they are also expected to treat their patients.

Callahan also feels that no person, physician or otherwise, "should have that kind of power over another, freely gained or not." The power to help a person die is truly enormous. But it is neither new nor excessive. It takes its place beside the power to replace a failing heart or kidney, or to decide not to. The physician is invested with the power to do whatever he or she thinks is in the best interest of the patient. As this power increases with medical progress, so does the responsibility to use it wisely, particularly when the decisions mean life or death. Serious risks are inherent in the patient-physician relationship. Although Callahan is in awe of such power and responsibility, many physicians live with both on a daily basis.

An important principle in medical ethics is beneficence: treatment and care should benefit the patient. In the context of assisted dying this principle fits between patient autonomy and paternalism. Beneficence leans toward patient autonomy if one agrees that the patient should decide when his suffering has gone on long enough, and toward paternalism if the physician is thought better equipped to make that decision. In general, when there is a difference of opinion, beneficence favors the physicians because of the ambiguity about what is best for the patient and who decides.

In a subtle form of paternalism, the physician guides her patient to the "correct" decision, often by stressing the positive aspects of a course of action while downplaying or even omitting relevant information concerning the negative aspects. Howard Brody recognizes the conflict between paternalism and patient autonomy as a manifestation of the power of the physician.[24] Not only do physicians often refuse to share their power with patients, they are often unaware how much power they have, or that it is even an issue.

The broad goals of medicine are to cure disease, to save and prolong life, and to relieve suffering. Usually these can all be met simultaneously. Kass sees a single goal of medicine, the preservation of health, with little room for the wants and desires of the patient.

The physician, he maintains, must remain true to this essential purpose and not be tempted by the demands of patients or society.[25] But this is much too narrow an assessment of the goals of medicine to suit most physicians and patients. When disease cannot be cured, relief of suffering becomes a primary objective. When relief of suffering includes the possibility of actually shortening life, the contradiction appears: shortening life is not prolonging life.

To resolve this conflict one or both of these goals must be modified and broadened. Prolonging life has already yielded to refusing or discontinuing treatment and to the ambiguity of the double effect. Relief of suffering is on the threshold of being expanded to include assisted dying. And why not? Many physicians agree that the interests of some patients should be met by earlier, more comfortable deaths. The executive editor of the *New England Journal of Medicine*, Marcia Angell, has pointed out in an editorial that "in such circumstances, it seems illogical and callous to acknowledge that a patient's interests may be best served by a peaceful death and then fastidiously to avoid helping to bring it about. The blanket proscription against shortening life is too rigid and limiting."[26] Diane Meier adds that "refusal to respond to a suffering patient's request for release is really an admission that the physician's ultimate obligation is not to the welfare of his patient. This refusal is at the very real cost of abandoning the patient to his sufferings in the name of rules and principles that can have very little meaning to the patient."[27] Even from a historical perspective, when a choice must be made between prolonging life and relieving suffering, the physician's primary responsibility is to relieve suffering. This is in the true tradition of medicine because our ability to significantly prolong life is a very recent development.

Another basic principle of medical ethics is nonmaleficence: do no harm. This has always been a relative principle because the practice of medicine often inflicts on patients discomfort or even pain, both of which are certainly forms of harm. The concept becomes far more complicated when it must be applied to life-sustaining treatment of patients with fatal diseases or to the role of the physician in helping the patient who wants to die. At this point the principles of helping and not harming the patient appear to come into conflict. When looked at more closely, however, particularly from the patient's point of view, these principles may overlap to the point of virtual agreement. Relief of intolerable suffering, be it from the disease itself or from the extremes of medical technology, must be weighed against earlier death. Many feel that unnecessary suffering, not death, is the ultimate harm and that compared with such suffering, early death is the lesser evil. Moreover, the competent patient should be in the best position to resolve this conflict. It should not be subject to empirical rulings by the medical profession or the state.

Concerned Ambivalence

Given the number of conflicting personal, professional, and moral pressures, it is small wonder that many physicians whose patients have fatal diseases are ambivalent about assisted dying. This range of thinking is reflected in the attitudes of the physicians interviewed, many of whom have been asked to assist in death in the past.

A neurologist noted that it is common for his patients to talk about assisted dying. "They hint at it, often in a half-joking manner, to sound you out or even to plan for the future. I see people all the time who are in terrible trouble, unable to breathe or to eat or to do much of anything, literally drowning in their own secretions. Their productive lives are over, they are suffering intensely, and they think they would be better off dead than alive. I could put myself in their shoes and say that if that was me, I would certainly think about it too."

Another neurologist had a similar perspective:

I have no objection to laws that would allow physicians under certain circumstances to be more active in helping people to die. It should be legal. I have seen patients over the years where it was blatantly obvious that they should have the ability to make these decisions. The alternative is foolish from every point of view; the patient, the family, the medical care cost, and so forth. It serves nobody's purpose to make these people live longer. We participate in a charade in which we are trying to maintain an individual purely because of some legal issues. I don't think it is even a moral issue at that point. It is an *immoral* issue. We are being forced to do this. It is quite common for the patient, as well as the family, to be in a sort of waiting mode, simply hoping that pneumonia or some other event will put an end to the situation.

A pulmonary disease specialist said

I take umbrage at the idea that physicians have no business in the issue of dying, that our job is only to save people. I think our job is much broader than that. I would favor a law where physicians would be allowed to play a direct role so that we could provide a safety net to the patient who is suffering. That's what patients worry about, and those are the questions they face. It also might be very useful for some patients to have an external, somewhat objective person, their physician, to help them think about these issues. I know that some physicians are going to shy away from this because they are afraid of the implications. It is just too scary. But some are ready to accept this role and others will grow into it.

Another pulmonary specialist felt differently: "It is partly my personal philosophy and partly my religious views, but I don't think that we should be in the business of helping people die. We are here to relieve suffering, but not at the cost of life. Death from pulmonary failure is slow and very uncomfortable but not truly painful. There is a lot of discouragement, and I would try to help with that. But life is rough all around and we have to deal with our losses and our difficulties. I try to find ways to help people cope with these problems."

A renal disease specialist said, "This opens up an issue not only for doctors but for all of society, as to what our values are around the end of life. I am troubled by a movement that equates care and helping patients at the end of their lives with laws that would enable doctors to provide lethal medications. While they may seem to be on a continuum, in the realm of our respect for life and what physicians' roles are in our society, they are very different."

A medical oncologist would refer a patient: "I have a lot of problems with legalization of assisted dying. I just think that physicians are supposed to be helping people, either by making them better or making them more comfortable. It would be a very bad mistake to blur the line and suddenly have them actively help people die. I wouldn't want to see physicians empowered to do that. If it were legal and a patient of mine wanted help in dying, I would say that there are physicians who don't feel the way I do and I would give them the names. I think there is a legitimate position on the other side. I just happen to disagree with it."

A medical oncologist separates practice from law: "If it were legal I would certainly help a person to take his own life. I already do that. If I think their decision is truly voluntary, I see it as my role to provide the help they ask for. However, I do not think that the law should be changed. For a small number of patients who would benefit from making it legal, the stance for the profession would be shifted."

A transplant surgeon observed, "There are unquestionably situations where it is appropriate to allow or even help somebody end unbearable suffering. The problem is how do you take that step without going too far? I truly believe that the individual ought to have jurisdiction over his or her own life, and in some cases even death. On theoretical grounds I have a lot of sympathy for that point of view and am probably supportive of it. On the other hand, could I carry it out in practice? I don't think I could."

Another testimony to some physicians' ambivalence is their personal double standard. Several of the physicians whom I interviewed clearly expected more comfortable deaths for themselves and their loved ones than they were willing to provide for patients. In essence they said, "I know exactly what I want for myself at the end of life, and how to get it. Would I provide that kind of help to my patients? Not a chance, until the law is changed."

Once the respect for human life is so low that an innocent person may be killed directly, even at his own request, compulsory euthanasia will necessarily be near. This could lead easily to killing all charity patients, the aged who are a public care, wounded soldiers, all deformed children, the mentally afflicted and so on. Before long the danger would be at the door of every citizen. *Bishop Joseph Sullivan*

I have gone forward, not as one travelling in a road cast up, but as a man walking through a miry place in which are stones here and there, safe to step on; but so situated that one step being taken, time is necessary to see where to step next. *John Woolman*

6
Public Concerns: Abuse and the Slippery Slope

There is understandable concern that legalization of assisted dying will entail risks, some immediate and realistic, others at the remote limits of imagination—medical error, abuse of vulnerable patients, legal extension of assisted dying beyond acceptable boundaries, financial pressure from public sources. Neither religious nor moral in origin, these issues are practical, pragmatic, and some say even predictable in nature. Taken to extremes, as they often intentionally are, they can be truly frightening. The prospect of moral disintegration to the level of the Holocaust of Nazi Germany is an exaggeration used primarily by those whose real objections are religious and moral but who realize that for wider appeal they must use arguments that are secular and more generally alarming than the threat of an afterlife of eternal damnation. These concerns are also hypothetical, with little or no basis in experience. They are therefore impossible to weigh and to evaluate in advance. Nevertheless, they

are the most troubling and cogent arguments against assisted dying
and must therefore be looked at very closely and objectively.

Physician Error

Physicians are not infallible, and the suggestion has been made that
people could decide to end their lives on the basis of an incorrect diagnosis or when the course of the disease and prognosis had not
been properly evaluated.[1] These are theoretical possibilities, but
they do not have much bearing on the patient who is dying. By the
time a person is dying of a chronic degenerative disease, the correct
diagnosis is almost self-evident. When someone on a respirator is dying of pulmonary failure, he clearly has pulmonary failure, and there
is little question about the underlying disease. The same is true for
renal failure and cancer and all of the other "bad" deaths we are
looking at.

Predicting the long-term outlook can be more complicated.
Estimating how long a person may live is approximate at best when
he still has several months to live, but forecasting becomes less difficult as the end draws near. Some chronic diseases, like multiple
sclerosis, are notorious for having remissions, but the trend is always
down. The experience of the physician and a record of the general
course of the individual patient are critical. The more variable the
course of the disease, the more important it is to be sure that further
remissions are unlikely and that death is near. Of the physicians interviewed in this study, the vast majority felt that lack of information
or understanding of the disease were not serious limitations; they
had confidence in their capacity to predict accurately for patients
with advanced disease. It is also important to be sure that all appropriate treatments that are acceptable to the patient have been
tried and have failed. The strongest voice, if not the last word, must
belong to the patient himself. He must feel free to discontinue or
refuse further treatment at any time.

Some worry that the physician may be unaware of a cure that

is just days away. This possibility is also remote. The time from laboratory to patient is measured in years rather than weeks, and information about new developments spreads rapidly in the medical world. Indeed, newspaper reports sometimes precede publication in medical journals. Furthermore, physicians have every reason to present their patients with the latest advances as soon as possible. The net result is that there are no potentially curative treatments that are unheard of today but will be ready for public use next week.

The statement that there is no such thing as an incurable disease may be a useful political claim by those who hope to wrest money for research from a skeptical government, but as a statement of medical fact it is tenuous at best. True, many potentially lethal diseases are curable early in their courses, but very rarely curable at the time of impending death. It is also said that no one can be sure that a situation is hopeless. There are no absolutes in medicine and seemingly miraculous recoveries or remissions can occur. Such miracles are too rare, however, to justify their inclusion in major medical decision-making processes. Although doctors cannot know absolutely what lies ahead, it is their professional responsibility to make well-educated guesses; forecasts that are beyond reasonable doubt. We accept or reject doctors' recommendations all the time, without routinely questioning whether or not they are correct. In so doing, we assume risks, even of death, or of permanent disability that may be worse than death. If doctors are to be held to extraordinary standards with respect to dying, they should be held to similar standards in all other aspects of medicine, and clearly they are not. Inability to know absolutely everything does not imply inability to know anything. The extent of this theoretical shortcoming should not be focused on assisted dying any more than it is on other serious end-of-life concerns. The risk that an airline flight may crash is very small but undeniable. Yet most of us fly without undue fear.

The patient, guided by his own philosophy, also has some responsibility in this interaction. The person who will endure untold suffering with the fervent expectation that tomorrow will bring a cure should not be discouraged. Someone who truly believes in miracles is unlikely to ask for assisted dying. On the other hand, the person who is suffering and dying today should not be required to endure prolongation of the process on the basis that the physician may be wrong. He must understand this minute theoretical risk and be willing to accept it, as is often the case when suffering is severe and life expectancy limited.

Another potential medical shortcoming is that physicians might be tempted to see assisted dying as an easy way out for themselves and to give up too soon. But everyone who acknowledges having done it, including some physicians in Holland who have participated in many assisted deaths, finds it a brutally stressful experience. None of the physicians whom I interviewed considered giving up too soon to be a significant possibility. All of them have experience with discontinuing treatment or supportive measures; some have even given narcotics in excess of what was necessary to relieve pain, thus bringing about earlier death. The decisions were made after all treatment had failed—at the far end of the management spectrum from giving up too soon. The acts, similar in many ways to assisted dying, were timely and compassionate.

The possibility of being asked to assist in dying might in fact make it harder for the physician to back away when curative treatment ended. Accepting a significant but troubling role at the end of life would encourage continued interest in all aspects of care before that. If a patient was suffering unreasonably, the physician would be obliged to share that suffering and to discuss the alternatives rather than turn the whole process over to someone else, such as a home hospice nurse.

Finally, the opportunity to give up sooner is already at hand. Far less troublesome than assisted dying is the earlier and easier step of withdrawing treatment, a practice that is done every day for appropriate patients. Yet this accepted and legal step has not in any way diminished the aggressive treatment practiced in our acute care hospitals. If withdrawing treatment is not considered to be an easy way out, assisted dying is even less likely to be.

Abuse

Assisted dying is a privilege sought by patients and acknowledged by much of the public and by many physicians as a desirable option. In a sense, assisted dying is itself a strategy of avoiding abuse—the abuse of being required to endure prolonged suffering. However badly laws that would permit assisted dying may be needed, like any others, they would be liable to evasion or violation. The term *abuse* implies that most of the time assisted dying would be legitimate and justifiable. Exceptions to this—early death urged on a patient by his family or physician, for example, or social pressure exerted on vulnerable patients—would constitute abuse. How common would this be? Those who cite the potential for abuse as a deterrent to legislation suggest that it would be commonplace and impossible to control. As we shall see later, both of these dangers are grossly exaggerated.

Before looking at specific aspects of the problem, it is important to put the entire prospect of abuse in perspective. How many people can we expect to be abused, and what would it mean? It is impossible to predict what the demand for assisted dying would be in this country. At first, legalization would certainly be confined to assisted suicide, which puts a great deal of responsibility on the patient. For physical and psychological reasons, this would limit the final act to a very small number of people, probably fewer than 1 percent of all deaths.[2]

Indeed, we have asked the wrong question about abuse. Given identical hypothetical circumstances, a fatal and painful illness with a life expectancy of four weeks, how many patients who are not being coerced in any way should be made to suffer unnecessarily to avoid the possibility of the wrongful early death of a single person who was persuaded by his family or physician—a hundred? five hundred? a thousand? Such violations cannot be completely prevented, but they would be rare. An important function of the law is to regulate these activities and reduce the risks to a minimum. The expected time that the patient in the above example would be deprived of is four weeks of intense suffering, hardly on the scale of the risk that society has accepted with criminal punishment, where we occasionally imprison people for years and even execute them for crimes that they did not commit. In short, in this country the number of patients requesting assisted suicide will probably be small and the risk of abuse smaller still. In addition, since most such people must have fatal diseases, associated with serious suffering and short life expectancies, the risk of abuse becomes both acceptable and manageable.

Family members are in an obvious position to apply pressure on a dying relative to end his or her life sooner. Reasons for this might include greed for an inheritance, exhaustion from prolonged and progressive caregiving, resentfulness of the burden that the illness is placing on the rest of the family, and malevolence, even hatred, toward the relative. Circumstances might force a family to take in an elderly but unwanted relative. Illness might aggravate the burden, and impending death might be more than the family was willing to deal with. Methods of exerting pressure range from simply making a person feel unwanted to dropping hints that life will be easier for the survivors when the person is gone to more aggressive persuasion, including pleading that it "really would be best for you and for all of us." Some families might even resort to ultimatums and threatening language or behavior.

The natural protection against this exceptional behavior is that most families are at least accommodating, if not loving and supporting, even under very difficult circumstances. Dysfunctional families often are not uniformly so. Families bent on abusing an ill relative have many outlets available short of encouraging suicide—withholding medical treatment, medications, or even adequate nutrition, for example. Furthermore, the family that wishes to shorten a relative's life can do it more safely alone, in the confines of their home. Trying to enlist the help of a physician creates a huge risk because she probably would not agree and might even notify the authorities that any mishap that might occur to the patient should be looked upon with suspicion. Indeed, the possibility of coercive abuse should be in the mind of any physician whose patient requests assisted dying and whose family seems to be encouraging it. The initial response of family members of a patient who makes such a request is usually just the opposite; they do not want their loved one to die any sooner than necessary. Some persuasion on the part of the patient is often required to gain even modest support. This clue might help to distinguish the typical family from the potentially abusive one. At some point, the physician should meet with the patient alone and ask appropriately probing questions concerning family attitudes, financial incentives, and the patient's own concept of himself as a burden on the family, and how the family may have influenced that concept.

The timetable of most terminal illness is such that a family would gain little by speeding up the process by a few days or weeks—certainly too little to make it worth any risk of detection. For the person who is elderly and terminally ill, life with an unloving and abusive family may in itself be reason enough to seek an early death. Bringing a physician into such a situation might even restore tranquillity and extend the life of the patient by making it possible to arrange for transfer to better surroundings. We already deal with similar problems when the families or surrogates of patients in coma seem inclined to discontinue supportive measures based on their own best interests rather than those of the patient. The competent, conscious patient at least has the possibility of speaking for himself. This is a risk that even the law is increasingly willing to take.

It is also possible, though unlikely in practice, that physicians might exert pressure on patients to elect earlier death. In its simplest form, this circumstance might arise from compassion carried too far, to the point of anticipating the patient's needs and even desires. The physician-ethicist Edmund Pellegrino has underscored this point: "When assisted suicide is legitimized, it places the patient at immense risk from the 'compassion' of others. Misdirected compassion in the foci of human suffering can be as dangerous as indifference."[3] Unfortunately, Pellegrino's rejection of assisted dying under any circumstances forces him to put absolute limits on compassion that are not shared by all physicians and certainly do not reflect or respect the best interests of many patients.

A second set of motives might involve the patient and his illness. Some patients are indeed demanding, unreasonable, and difficult for their physicians to deal with. Such people, however, are unlikely candidates for mischievous persuasion because rather than being docile and malleable, they are usually very strong willed. As such, they are the least likely to heed any suggestion concerning shortening of life. On the other hand, fatigue, burnout, and frustration over failure to control a patient's disease might weigh on the physician, perhaps to the point of seeking an easy way out. Assisted dying could conceivably become impersonal and routine, even a route for resolving all life-and-death problems that refuse to yield to other treatment. The possibility exists that some physicians, for personal or political reasons, would become "euthanasia enthusiasts," immoderately active and insufficiently selective.[4]

Finally, one must not overlook the truly malevolent physician who takes it upon herself to rid her practice or the world of unwanted people. This monster—who should be confined to the notoriety of horrific film and literature—might euthanize a patient to cover up some error in medical treatment. But most serious medical mishaps occur in hospitals, where they are open to scrutiny and would be hard to cover up simply by eliminating the victim. If a large amount of money were involved, a greedy family might "buy" an equally greedy physician, persuading her to circumvent the objections of the patient. The most ghastly image is of the physician whose quest for power culminates in the taking of life. As Richard Doerflinger has written, "Human beings are tempted to enjoy exercising power over others; ending another person's life is the ultimate exercise of that power. . . . The skill and the instinct to kill are more easily turned to other lethal tasks once they have an opportunity to exercise themselves."[5] The hunter-killer instinct latent in all mankind supposedly surfaces with the first taste of blood, overcoming all restrictions imposed by culture, civilization, humanity, and education. But even if such physicians do exist outside literature, no law against assisted dying would have any effect on their quest for blood.

When a person is suffering and dying, the physician may increase the dose of morphine at the request of the patient or the family, or on her own initiative, bringing life to a gradual or even abrupt end. This is done frequently, and is well within the law. It would be far more cumbersome and risky for the physician to try to persuade the patient to take his own life. The physician is seen by some to have extraordinary powers of suggestion, even to the extent of being able to persuade patients to accept measures that would shorten their lives. Undeniably, the social and professional role of the physician and the dependence forced on patients by illness effect a very unequal relationship. But this is true of every decision-making process involving physician and patient, including those of life and death. In general, shortening the life of a patient is counterproductive for the physician, who is paid for taking care of living patients and whose source of payment disappears when the patient dies.

Society has a moral and legal responsibility to protect its weaker members from mistreatment. Opponents of assisted dying fear that some people would be particularly vulnerable to abuse. The aged, the infirm, the disabled, the poor, minorities, and even women are cited as vulnerable groups—more than half the population. Furthermore, these categories of vulnerability are cumulative. But we should recognize that vulnerability does not apply equally to all members of the groups listed above, nor is it confined to them. An elderly impoverished black woman who is seriously ill with cancer may succeed in getting the medical care she chooses while a much younger wealthy Caucasian male who has AIDS may be vulnerable and at the mercy of the health care system. Some critics consider it self-evident that every person in these vulnerable groups would be at greatly increased risk of being pushed into early deaths. Such abuse would be directed at particular patients not for personal reasons but simply because they are weak and vulnerable and more easily manipulated. On an individual basis, this would represent abuse; on a societal basis, it would epitomize the slippery slope. The issue is extremely important and deserves close analysis.

In practice, the result of vulnerability is far more apt to be neglect than undue attention. Indeed, the common characteristic that can render members of these several groups vulnerable is inability to get what they want or need to make their lives more bearable. Neglect has many faces and is in no way confined to medical care. It extends to every aspect of social need—food, clothing, shelter, education, employment, and general access to the many opportunities and advantages that give quality to life. To be vulnerable is to risk being bypassed by society. The related question is why social neglect would necessarily lead vulnerable people to want or accept assisted dying. Who would gain by promoting the earlier death of a person who is already dying? Certainly, if conditions were bad enough, with a wretched life compounded by a fatal disease, the patient himself might see it that way and might wish to die. But if the wretched life antedated the disease by many years, it would be hard to say that the life itself had now tipped the balance and that it, rather than the fatal disease, was the major motive. Poor people can be very sick, too.

The ultimate source of abuse of the vulnerable would have to be physicians. Yet in a society that virtually sanctions medical neglect of many people, one has good reason to ask why a physician would bother to abuse them. To abuse the vulnerable, physicians would have to greatly exceed the role allotted them by an uncaring society and assume responsibility for the deaths of people that they don't even know, performing a task that most consider to be stressful and odious, at best. Indeed, the vulnerable patient rarely has any one person in the entire system whom he can call his doctor. It is hard to believe that anyone would help a patient to die because he was wretchedly poor and not because he was already dying from a painful cancer that was beyond treatment. It is equally incredible that a medical system that has found it expedient to neglect so many would suddenly change its mind and offer them the latest and most controversial in all of medical interventions.

On the contrary, the vulnerable will remain at the low end of the spectrum of medical care.[6] The poor and uninsured are the least likely to have an ongoing relationship with a physician that would lead to assisted dying, even if it were entirely appropriate. Among the impoverished and otherwise vulnerable, most of those who would request assisted dying because of serious illness would suffer the same distress and have just as good reasons for their requests as anybody else. Yet we may well go through a phase where their legitimate requests are denied, even when legal, because they are among the vulnerable.

A vast oversimplification is the argument by Yale Kamisar that lack of universal access to adequate medical care, and therefore to good pain control, is the central problem, and that when it is solved the desire for assisted dying will disappear. According to this stance, society should attack the conditions of poverty long before agreeing with patients that early death may be desirable.[7] But the desire for assisted dying and access to health care are entirely separate issues. Many forms of suffering other than poorly controlled pain cause people to request assisted dying, and comprehensive health care cannot prevent "bad deaths." Although a regrettably large number of Americans do not have adequate health care insurance or coverage, the vast majority are receiving the best care available anywhere in the world. Among those who do have good health care are some who suffer significantly at the end of life and who, regardless of their other options, would still prefer earlier, more comfortable deaths. These are people who understand the current health care system, who benefit from it, and who are still most openly concerned about how their lives may end. They are also the most likely to get the help they want. It seems completely inappropriate to hold assisted dying up until we have total health care, not to mention the elimination of poverty. One can hardly say to the dying, "It is too bad that you are suffering, but some people aren't getting adequate health care."

Prevention of Abuse

To minimize the risk of abuse, requirements and guidelines have been proposed by every group advocating assisted dying. Because these will be essential for the development of equitable and responsible laws, they require close examination. The following analysis compares suggested guidelines from many sources, including the Dutch experience, the referenda of Washington, California, and Oregon, numerous proposals in state legislatures, and several thoughtful academic individuals and groups.[8]

THE PATIENT

The patient must be conscious and competent, the criteria for which we have examined elsewhere. Much proposed legislation incorporates a requirement that the illness be in a terminal stage, with a life expectancy of less than six months. This is an arbitrary figure that is not universally applicable. Clearly the person who is far advanced in his illness may have an outside life expectancy measured in hours or days instead of months. Many people die within a day or two of arriving at hospice, and the average time before death at Connecticut Hospice is only about two weeks.

The farther away the terminal event, the harder it is to predict its timing; arguing about six months is trivial and misleading. Most people who have fatal illnesses do not want to shorten their lives by nearly that long. In Holland many patients begin to discuss assisted dying far in advance but activate the process much later, within a few weeks or even days of the expected time of death from the disease. Just having the option of assisted dying may encourage a patient to endure longer, even to the natural end of life, knowing that help is available if wanted. As palliative care at home continues to improve, more people will put off exercising their option for assisted dying until they are near death and relief has failed. On the other hand, there is no limit to how far in advance a person can initiate discussion about assisted dying. It can take place as soon as a diagnosis is made, or when it becomes clear that the illness will probably be fatal. This early dialogue alerts the physician that an actual request may be forthcoming at some later date. The more frequently assisted dying is reviewed, the less chance for misunderstanding between patient and physician as to the duration and sincerity of the request.

As we have seen, for a small but important group of people, primarily those with neurological diseases, suffering is great but the illnesses are slowly progressive, making six months a meaningless figure. These are people who may endure suffering that in every way justifies assisted dying, but who have life expectancies of much more than six months.[9] Eventually, laws permitting assisted dying should accommodate these people.

To be a candidate for assisted dying, the patient must be enduring what he considers to be intolerable suffering. Pain and other forms of suffering are subjective sensations that can be described but cannot be measured. Others can confirm that the patient has a horrible disease, but only the patient can determine the limits of what he is willing to endure. To do so he must be informed of the exact nature of his diagnosis and prognosis and of all of the alternatives available, including comfort care and hospice. He must have received or rejected all other treatments.

THE REQUEST

A patient-initiated request for assisted dying is very different from the usual presentation of treatment options by a physician, with the patient giving consent to some chosen treatment. No one should *consent* to have his life shortened. Once assisted dying is legalized, its availability will be common knowledge. If in the course of discussing terminal care a patient asks what all his options are, assisted dying should certainly be included among them. The actual request, however, must originate with the patient. It must be voluntary and free of any coercion by family or physician. For purposes of documentation, it should be in writing and witnessed by at least one person who knows the patient but has no financial interest in his death.

Not only must a voluntary request come from a person who is competent and informed, but it should be a durable request that expresses the person's continuing resolve. Most suggested legislation has required a two-week waiting period to allow the patient to consult others and to consider and reconsider his options. To provide help too quickly would court the possibility of an impetuous act at a time of unusual stress or disappointment. To insist upon too long a waiting period would subject the person to more of the very unnecessary suffering he has sought to escape. The opposite side of durability is revocability: the person can rescind his request at any time. When the method of death is assisted suicide, the patient has the greatest possible control.

PHYSICIANS

The physician's first responsibility is to ascertain that the request originated with the patient and is truly autonomous, and that the patient is competent to make major medical and life-and-death decisions. It is incumbent on the physician to make sure that the patient understands the nature of his illness, how far his disease has progressed, what various possible scenarios lie ahead, and what all the options are, including assisted dying. The patient should be required to weigh carefully the irreversibility of an earlier death against his current level of suffering, his probable future suffering, and some reasonable estimate of the expected duration of the process. Except for confidential conversations about family attitudes, this discussion should probably take place in the presence of a member of the family, assuming that the patient agrees. Furthermore, the discussion should be ongoing, spread over two or three visits. The patient should have every opportunity to review these salient points.

A long-standing relationship with the physician is ideal but should not be required. It is not even required in Holland, though it is typical there.[10] Such a relationship can be a strong deterrent to coercion by the family. In the presence of serious and prolonged illness, it is unusual for a physician to know a patient well but not know some family members. Although a specialist does not have the advantage of the family physician, who may have visited the patient at home, she may still have a clear picture of patient-family interaction.

It is important for patients and the public to understand the physician's pivotal position in this relationship. The patient can request but cannot demand assisted dying. The physician can agree or not agree in principle, and can decide when to provide the help requested. Going to a second physician is exceedingly difficult if the first physician turns down the request for any valid reason other than personal unwillingness to assist in dying. If she is personally opposed to assisted dying and will not provide help, she should make her position clear as soon as the subject comes up. If she is willing to help, she has a similar obligation.

Independent evaluation of the patient is a fundamental step for avoiding abuse. Second or even third medical opinions should come from physicians who are not close associates of the primary physician and who do not know the patient. The second physician should accept in principle the concept of physician-assisted dying for some patients but should be experienced enough to ask appropriate questions of the patient and family: How did the idea of early death arise in this case? Has pressure been exerted for or against assisted death by the primary physician or the family? Do the patient and his family fully comprehend the nature of the illness? How far has the disease progressed? And what are the patient's short- and long-term outlooks? All alternative courses should be discussed, and assisted dying should be placed in its appropriate perspective. The resolve of the patient should be questioned closely. Some form of psychological evaluation should be available at the request of either physician in order to rule out treatable depression. I do not believe that such evaluation should be required, though some states may mandate it. Suggestions have been made that requests for assisted dying should be reviewed by ombudsmen or even ethics committees. These cumbersome requirements could provide review of the paperwork but would shed little light on the competence of the patient and the voluntariness of the request. Such vital information can only come through personal interviews.

FAMILY

If there is increased safety in having two or more physicians involved with a request for assisted dying, there is even more to be gained by including members of the family. Although some people may prefer that all family members be excluded, it should be pointed out that it is in the interests of the patient to include family members in their discussions. Family involvement also offers significant protection to the physician. Close family members usually sit in on conversations between patients and physicians concerning proposed treatment, particularly when serious risks are involved. It helps the patient to have someone else receive the same information so that they can review it together at a later time. Never would this be more important than in any discussion of assisted dying with a physician. The best protection against abuse is having close family members and two physicians all agree with the patient that assisted death is a reasonable option. Regardless of whether the family is supportive of a patient's decision, a physician would be unlikely to risk exerting even the most subtle pressure in the presence of a family member. If the patient agreed, even discussion of family attitudes could take place in the presence of relatives. Nothing would discourage a family more from exerting undue pressure on a patient than the realization that the physician was alert to such a possibility.

DOCUMENTATION AND REPORTING

Two other steps designed to prevent abuse are documentation and reporting. Documentation of the entire interaction, beginning with the first suggestion by the patient and concluding with the circumstances surrounding the death, should be in the patient's record, either in the physician's office or at the hospital or both. This should include the formal request by the patient, summaries of any interviews with the patient and the family, and a formal letter from the secondary physician and/or psychiatrist. The major purpose of documentation is to establish the fact that the request for assisted dying was initiated by the patient and that he was well informed and competent and could explain his reasons appropriately. Recording the request on videotape would add a layer of legal protection for the family and physician.

Closely related to documentation is reporting of the death to the coroner or the state medical association, or some other designated office. The coroner already must receive a death certificate, and it would be appropriate to list physician-assisted dying as one of the causes of death. The potential stigma of suicide would be reduced by listing the patient's fatal disease first and assisted dying second. If the patient requested and was given a lethal medication for assisted suicide, that should be listed as one of the causes of death, though it might not be known whether the patient took the drugs or died of the underlying disease.

In the first stages of legally integrating assisted dying into medical practice, it will be essential to have information on all patients who request and are granted assistance. A formal report could be submitted to the state medical association or some representative body for collation and analysis. The report might include the name of the physician, the place of death, the insurance carrier, and demographic information about the patient (including race, age, gender, and physical disability); the nature and duration of the disease and previous treatment, including pain control; the nature and the extent of the patient's suffering and alternative treatments offered; names of other physicians involved, as well as witnesses and family members involved with the request; and a copy of the written request itself. Only through documentation and reporting will it be possible to evaluate any safeguards that are adopted. Several writers have decried the fact that "safeguards have not been adequately tested and shown to be effective" and that "no one has the essential empirical information. . . . The question is too important to resolve without data."[11] These critics overlook the fact that the only way to obtain reliable and objective data relative to our own society will be to take the significant step of legalizing assisted dying in a few states. Then we can determine which safeguards are necessary and which are not and whether others are put at significant risk when we accommodate the needs of the dying and those who would help them.

Collection of data would make it possible to review the practice of assisted dying in the first states to do so, providing important information for the rest of the country. Over time these data would reveal the frequency of assisted deaths provided by individual physicians, in individual institutions or nursing homes, and under the auspices of certain HMOs or health care plans, as well as other details, like the financial status of the patients and families. As a byproduct, the collection of such data would not only make it possible to initiate steps to detect abuse but would serve notice to potential abusers that detection was possible.

Finally, there is absolutely no way of knowing in advance whether the large categories of people classified as vulnerable would desire early death or would try, for inappropriate reasons, to influence physicians to provide them with such. It will be incumbent on us to examine the issue of vulnerability within our own divergent population, and Oregon presents an opportunity to do so. Very basic information would quickly establish whether the preponderance of requests and fulfilled assisted deaths are among the seemingly vulnerable members of our society.

One might ask why the doctor should report assisted death at all? Even though it is required, only about half of the assisted deaths in Holland are reported. Although laws regulating assisted dying could certainly require that reports be filed, with reasonable penalties for not doing so, another more pressing legal reality exists in this country: the risk of lawsuit by the family or even other caregivers. One could make the physician's immunity to such prosecution depend on having prepared and filed the appropriate reports. The presence of signed reports could preempt the process, establishing the patient's autonomy in directing his own death. The inclusion of other supportive people, such as family members, would further strengthen the evidence of the reports.

It is important to note that the potential for all these abuses already exists but is widely accepted and is not considered to be of great concern. Withholding or withdrawing treatment can be done at the request of the patient or of the family. As we have seen, in some cultures and situations, family and physician may even make a decision for a patient who could perfectly well decide for himself. Finally, in appropriate situations physicians occasionally withhold or withdraw treatment on their own, with little or no discussion with the family. In spite of these accepted freedoms and minimal safeguards, withholding and withdrawing treatment have not resulted in wholesale abuse and are legitimate options for patients, families, and physicians.

The steps that could be taken to prevent abuse are so numerous that it is possible too many safeguards could be implemented—so many that the terminal patient might not live long enough to get through the process, even if he has the strength and the money. Many who object to physician-assisted dying in principle will never be satisfied and will continue to introduce layers of potential abuse, requesting additional safeguards. As two opponents have promised,

"We morally oppose euthanasia and physician-assisted suicide and would continue that opposition even if adequate legal safeguards could be developed."[12]

The Slippery Slope

Beyond the opposition to assisted dying based on concern about potential abuse is the threat of the so-called slippery slope. According to this theory, legalization of voluntary assisted dying, which in itself might be harmless, would be followed by nonvoluntary euthanasia, involving patients whose current personal desires could not be evaluated. From there it would be a short step to involuntary euthanasia, where death was forced upon people who understood perfectly well what was going on and did not want to die. This practice could be expanded in any direction, to eliminate the incompetent, the elderly, the disabled, racial minorities—any group that society deemed to be an unwanted burden. The endpoint would be a moral Holocaust reminiscent of Nazi Germany. As Edmund Pellegrino puts it, "Euthanasia and assisted suicide are socially disastrous. They are not containable by placing legal limits on their practice. Arguments to the contrary, the slippery slope is an inescapable, logical, psychological, historical and empirical reality."[13]

Some proponents of this theory believe that voluntary assisted dying may sometimes be justifiable and acceptable but that full legalization carries too great a risk for society. Others oppose even the first step, usually on moral or religious grounds, and postulate the entire sequence for emphasis and broader appeal. Both groups present the sequence as being inevitable and unstoppable. Doerflinger writes, "Removal of the taboo against assisted suicide will lead to destructive expansions of the right to kill the innocent . . . opening what may be a Pandora's Box of social evils."[14] Once on the slope, our society would be unable to escape the abyss of Nazi Germany. A line could neither be drawn nor held that would confine the harm that we would do to ourselves. The obvious conclusion is that the end is so horrible and so certain that it is much safer not to take the initial step, even if it would benefit a substantial number of people: "There are no good moral reasons to limit euthanasia once the principle of taking life for that purpose has been legitimated," writes Daniel Callahan. "If we really believe in self determination, then any competent person should have the right to be killed by a doctor for any reason that suits him. If we believe in relief of suffering, then it seems to be cruel and capricious to deny it to the incompetent. There is in short no reasonable or logical stopping point once the turn is made down the road to euthanasia, which could easily turn into a convenient and commodious expressway."[15]

The slippery slope is a public concern that needs to be examined much more closely than it usually is. Presented by some as a precipitous decline, plunging inevitably downward, the "slope" is quite different if we can look at it as a series of steps. Hard-core opponents of assisted dying cannot see it this way, of course; they consider the smallest step hazardous, if only by implication. Others who are less doctrinaire, though, agree that some steps near the top are on level ground and are eminently safe, while others near the bottom are indeed precarious. Those who favor assisted dying believe that a secure landing can be maintained on that stairway, and they have opinions about how far down that landing should be built.

The slippery slope has been described as having two components, logical and psychological.[16] The logical component dictates that if we accept assisted dying, we are committed to accepting other practices that we do not approve of, and that we cannot escape from this commitment. A rational boundary will move, if it exists at all. With no logical reason to halt an unacceptable progression, we should not take the first step, however humane and reasonable it may seem. In the psychological phase the attitudes of physicians and the public toward the value of life would be eroded, resulting in greater acceptance of violence and murder, as well as a broadening of the range of what people found "acceptable" for assisted dying. Once assisted dying is deemed appropriate for some people, the criteria would be extended, and killing would be approved for other reasons.

Indeed, although the line between allowing a patient to die and any form of assisted dying is essential to much religious and moral theory and has been invoked in several court decisions, it is indistinct in much of today's ethical thinking and in clinical usage, blurred by the practice of discontinuing any and all treatment at the patient's request and by the use of large doses of narcotics, with their easily obscured double effect. But the distinction between physician-assisted suicide and voluntary euthanasia is more easily seen. In all likelihood, the first laws that will be passed in any states to permit assisted dying will be limited to assisted suicide. As we have seen, the advantages and disadvantages of this limitation include the high degree of patient responsibility, the low potential for abuse, and greater acceptability by the medical profession and lawmakers than for euthanasia. Such laws would unfairly exclude the small group of people who were physically unable to ingest medications. On the other hand, sophisticated suicide devices could be devised that could be activated by any but the totally disabled person. The question then would be how much technical help the physician is allowed provide and still leave the ultimate responsibility up to the patient, thereby avoiding the stigma of euthanasia. Eventually, in the name of equality, the courts would practically be required to broaden the concept of physician-assisted dying to include active euthanasia by the physician, at least for some patients. This transition is so predictable and reasonable that it should not in any way be considered a step along the slippery slope, though inevitably some will label it that.

My personal feeling is that assisted dying should ultimately include both assisted suicide and euthanasia and that the patient and physician together will be in the best position to decide what is most appropriate. This would permit the inclusion of people who are suffering severely, meet all other accepted criteria for assisted dying, and can take oral medication but for psychological reasons prefer to have more direct help. My own interviews and the Dutch experience indicate that many people would prefer euthanasia over assisted suicide if they had a choice. This, too, is a predictable step that should not be seen as a slide on the slippery slope.

The next distinction is between voluntary euthanasia and nonvoluntary euthanasia of people who are not competent. The line here prohibiting nonvoluntary euthanasia should be generally established and respected. With experience and thoughtful consideration, however, one significant exception should eventually be allowed: the person who anticipates dementia. Such a person would have to plan ahead for nonvoluntary euthanasia by making an advance directive while still competent. The legal requirements for providing assisted dying for any noncompetent patients would be very complicated and would require close scrutiny by the courts. However far off such a possibility may be, it should not be totally discarded as a perilous step.

The lives and deaths of people with dementia, who are neither in coma nor dependent on any removable life-support systems, have already been the subject of considerable commentary.[17] The importance of extending assisted dying to some who are noncompetent lies in the large numbers of people who can expect to have Alzheimer's disease as our population ages. Among the many who fear this disease will be a few who are farsighted enough to wish to avoid the indignity of total dementia and brave enough to undertake the necessary planning. Our laws and practices should find a way to accommodate these people. Indeed, our courts have already moved ahead in this controversial area by respecting the past wishes of patients now in coma to have artificial support withdrawn.

Families can already make significant decisions concerning the lifesaving use or nonuse of antibiotics for relatives who are incompetent and reside in nursing homes and who develop acute infections. Unfortunately, nursing homes often do not request clear directives from responsible relatives, nor do they necessarily heed such directives at the time of decision making. Most also lack close supervision by physicians. As a result, patients are often sent to the emergency room of the nearest hospital for any acute problems. Treatment is initiated, even when the family would prefer a more timely "natural" death.

Finally, the line on involuntary euthanasia should be firmly established and maintained. The door to all the atrocities and horrors envisioned on a slippery slope hinges on involuntary euthanasia. And all arguments to the contrary, there is no practical reason to believe that acceptance of voluntary euthanasia would inevitably lead to involuntary euthanasia. The most important boundary—the difference between volition and coercion—is difficult neither to define nor to recognize or understand. Any physician or family member can distinguish between a person who is suffering and wants to die and one who, though suffering, wants to live. A continuing request for death speaks for itself. A patient who does not want help in dying will not bring up the subject. If it is brought up by someone else, he will reject it. To be a candidate for euthanasia, a patient must be fatally ill, be suffering significantly, and request assisted death— three criteria that may be overlooked on purpose but are hard to escape by accident. We are in no way doomed to a "social drift" from voluntary to involuntary euthanasia.

In summary, I believe that physician-assisted dying eventually should be extended to include not only assisted suicide but also voluntary euthanasia. Nonvoluntary euthanasia is generally unacceptable but should eventually be granted one exception: the patient who made his wishes clear in advance, when he was fully competent. Involuntary euthanasia should never be allowed. I also feel that for purposes of comparison of different degrees of incline on the slope, the entire end-of-life spectrum should be reviewed. It is pragmatic at this time to speak only of assisted suicide, but it is also misleading if one believes that assisted dying should eventually include euthanasia. Furthermore, these two activities are too close together in theory and practice to be distinguished on the so-called slope. Indeed, the slope is nearly level ground up to the precipice of involuntary euthanasia. By establishing a safety fence a few feet from the edge in specific cases, one can even stand safely on the narrow ledge of nonvoluntary euthanasia.

Some in society are trained to kill but required to keep these activities within strict bounds. Soldiers must transform themselves from professional killers to peacekeepers or even civilians abruptly and completely.[18] They may have psychological scars from their war experiences, but only a very few suffer a permanent breakdown of their respect for life, nor does the existence of a military cause such a breakdown in society. Police, though not actually trained to kill, are licensed to do so, either to protect others or in self-defense. But this license is not unrestricted, and police who use deadly force are routinely required to justify their actions. There is no reason why voluntary physician-assisted dying should be any more dangerous than these widely accepted exceptions to society's proscription against killing.

The hypothesis of the slippery slope overlooks the role that physicians would have to play in the transformation. They would have to lead the way onto such a slope. But there is nothing to indicate that, once authorized to help people die, they would be carried away with this activity. A slide into moral oblivion could not result from the misbehavior of a few rogue physicians. It would require a change in the attitude of the entire profession, including the AMA. The AMA does not discuss this possibility because its leaders do not believe that it could happen. Their statement that "the societal risks of involving physicians in medical interventions to cause patients' death is too great in this culture to condone euthanasia or assisted suicide at this time" places the responsibility on our society and culture and overlooks the leading role that the medical profession and the AMA would have to play.[19] The act of assisting in death is far too challenging for the medical profession to embrace in a reckless fashion. The AMA is a conservative organization that will resist legalized assisted dying up to a point, but I believe that it will eventually modify its position and accept some responsibility for helping its members adjust to the more complicated roles that society expects of them.

NAZI GERMANY

The bottom of the slippery slope is often characterized as the Holocaust of Nazi Germany. After the war, an American physician used Hitler's genocide to attack early thoughts of euthanasia in this country.[20] While the Nazis had used euthanasia to give their practices a veneer of acceptability, Leo Alexander reversed the reasoning and used the history of Nazi atrocities to make euthanasia unacceptable. Although the horror of the Holocaust is etched in the minds of most people, the slippery slope leading down to it had no relation to voluntary assisted dying.[21] Indeed, there was no slope at all. Shortly after coming to power in 1933, the Nazis passed a law on Prevention of Hereditarily Ill Offspring. This provided compulsory sterilization for patients who were mentally retarded or who had serious genetic defects. This was followed by the Children's Action, decreed by Hitler to identify "all severe cases of idiocy, mongoloidism, microcephalic disorders, hydrocephaly, deformed extremities, and paralysis." Upon the agreement of a committee of three physicians, the children were moved to special pediatric wards, where they were euthanized without parental knowledge or consent. Shortly after the beginning of the war similar wards were set up for patients in mental hospitals, to eliminate those who were considered unfit for work after at least five years of protective care. Again the families were never notified. The secret of this program was badly kept, and when churches protested, the direct killing of mental patients stopped. Many, however, were allowed to die of starvation in the ensuing years.

 The Nazi corruption of euthanasia bore no resemblance to the original meaning of the word, nor to its use today in the concept of assisted dying. They sought to whitewash and legitimize the process of eliminating "defective" members of society by deliberately misusing the word. Under Hitler, the government decided who would die, why, when, and how. There were no choices on the parts of the victims or their families. Sterilization and death were far from voluntary. The value of life was determined by the state, not the individual. The actual places of death were hidden, and the causes were attributed to such diseases as heart failure and pneumonia.

The Nazi atrocities were the brainchild of one individual and the work of people who consciously repudiated the humane and humanitarian approaches to ethics of the entire Western world. It was no step at all to move on to the deliberate extermination of all whom the Nazis considered to be subhuman forms of life—gypsies, Jews, homosexuals, and many people of Slavic origin. Mass extermination in Germany did not grow out of their earlier euthanasia program. The seeds for extermination of Jews were sown long before, in an atmosphere of vicious racism, and were destined to bear bitter fruit even if there had been no program for euthanasia. One can hardly say that Nazi Germany progressed down a slippery slope when the publication of *Mein Kampf* and the acceptance of its author as the country's leader placed it at the bottom of any such slope right from the beginning.

It was a black mark on German medicine, at one time the envy of the entire world, that physicians participated in these activities. A critical boundary was crossed between healing and killing, and "the medicalization of killing—the imagery of killing in the name of healing, was crucial to that terrible step."[22] Doctors who had the stomach to terminate the lives of mentally incompetent or deranged people were selected to help design and run the death camps. Fifteen were convicted at the war crimes trials at Nuremberg, and seven were sentenced to death. Why so many physicians knowingly participated in such atrocities is not known. Some undoubtedly wished to curry favor with the Nazi Party. Others may have felt threatened or overwhelmed by the immense power of the party and feared for their own safety. It must be recalled that the physicians were not alone in being corrupted under the regime. The legal profession of Germany was similarly overwhelmed, as was the ministry. The

Catholic Church, not only in Germany but also in Rome, asked few questions and said very little about what was going on inside Nazi Germany.

AMERICAN SOCIETY

The slippery slope argument now suffers from overuse, having been applied to birth control, abortion, advance directives, DNR orders, and removal of life support. The threat of abortion was that it would lead not only to devaluation of life but to infanticide. It has clearly done neither. Because both birth control and abortion would be forced upon minorities, it was said that they would lead to racial genocide. Again, the poor and minorities are now less apt to have access to either of these than are other members of society. Some activities that were previously sharply criticized, such as advance directives and removal of life support, are now deemed acceptable and even desirable by the same people who originally objected to them. One is forced to conclude not only that the original predictions were wrong but that the thinking leading up to them was also mistaken, if not deliberately misleading.

The slippery slope has been a graphic slogan for many causes. But what would be required to make assisted dying the start of such a slope? Certainly not a few errant physicians. The push would have to be much more forceful to initiate the complete reversal of our moral and legal commitment as a nation. Some cataclysm would have to occur whereby our entire society plunged into the abyss, deciding as a matter of public policy that large groups of our own citizens were no longer desirable and should be eliminated. Every step of the way would have to be legally sanctioned, and publicly accepted, if not actually applauded. Every person who seriously thinks that assisted dying would put us on a slippery slope should acknowledge now that he or she could personally approve of the extermination of the elderly, of blacks, of the weak and defenseless. For without such consent, culturewide, there can be no plunge down the slope. Such a moral reversal, if it were possible, would hardly be influenced by puny laws against assisted dying. Nazi Germany had perfectly good laws against murder, laws that applied to some but in no way interfered with the atrocities dealt out to others. While clearly not beyond the imaginations of some, I submit that such changes in our society are totally beyond reason. Certainly this is not the direction that the United States is taking or is likely to take. Our society is moving steadily toward greater tolerance and respect for individual rights, some of which were unthinkable until very recently. Interracial marriages are protected by law. Regulations prohibiting discrimination against homosexuals in the job market are moving into place, and the notion of legal marriage between homosexuals has even begun to gain support. Moreover, U.S. international policy often suggests that we are holding ourselves up, whether rightly or not, as a model of human rights for the world.

Nothing on the horizon suggests that our society is in any danger of reversing itself morally. Yet the threat of a slippery slope implies that the continued suffering of a few elderly, pitiful people at the end of life is all that stands between us and total moral disintegration. These unfortunate people must live out their final days in agony, or sedated into oblivion, in order to save our children and their children from becoming social monsters, or the victims of social monsters. Sparing people unnecessary suffering is a strange way of devaluing life. We are, in fact, a society that needs greater acceptance of death and dying, not in violence but in peace. Peaceful death with the help of compassionate physicians is exactly the opposite of suffering the violence of uncontrolled disease. Physician-assisted dying would put a good and visible face on some deaths that would otherwise be horrible.

Not only are we balancing the rights of those who now wish to die against those in the future who may not, but we are saying that the possible abrogation of rights in the future outweighs the clear violation of the rights of current victims of disease.[23] A society that prohibits assisted death to a suffering person and another society that puts to death those who are burdensome have one serious defect in common. Both are placing society's interest far ahead of the freedom of the individual. In doing so, they are equally mistaken and equally dangerous. A society that through guidelines and laws focuses on the rights and interests of the individual, now and in the future, can avoid both of these mistakes by respecting the needs of those who wish to die as well as those who do not.[24]

Health Care Financing

A final major area of public concern is the financing of medical care and its potential effect on assisted dying. Some see health care financing as the ice on the slope. In fact, it is an altogether separate issue, one of great complexity in its own right.

The United States is often castigated for not having a comprehensive health care delivery system, and some feel that legalized assisted dying would be used as a form of cost containment and therefore should not even be considered until a better system is in place. "The paramount reason for euthanasia is neither patient dignity nor relief of patient suffering, but saving money; not the patient's interests but those of society," writes one critic.[25] The financial structure of our health care system compares poorly with that of most other countries of the Western world. Attempts at comprehensive change have failed, and incremental changes are evolving very slowly. But physician-assisted dying is a separate issue from financing health care and will have little or no effect on the likelihood or urgency of developing a more responsible health delivery system. In the meantime, the issue of physician-assisted dying should not be held hostage to the complicated problem of health care financing.

Resources to pay for medical treatment and for research will always be scarce. Competition persists between preventive medicine for the healthy, acute and chronic care of the ill, and medical research for future care. Even countries that provide universal health care must make choices and set limits. Changing our health care system will benefit those who are currently excluded, but it will do nothing to lessen the total cost or the need for measures to control costs. I do not believe, however, that these measures will ever include the promotion of assisted dying for economic reasons.

We have seen the financial burden that serious illness can place on patients and families. To analyze the larger issue we must go beyond the immediate family and see who would benefit financially and who would lose by earlier deaths.[26] The health care system in the United States is undergoing rapid change, and the direction and the final point of equilibrium are not yet clear. Until recently the financial interests of all involved in delivering health care were obvious and easily understood; most of the medical care system reflected the interests of the patient. Publicly the patient's well-being remains the dominant theme, but everyone, including patients themselves, now wonders whether policy continues to reflect this concern. The roles of physicians, hospitals, and other health care providers are no longer clear. As people began to live longer and the capacity of medicine to treat illness expanded, expenditures rose unchallenged, and the entire health industry took advantage of it. The institution of managed care to control costs is changing every aspect of this dynamic.

Insurance companies and health maintenance organizations (HMOs) are increasingly responsible for managing the finances of much of the nation's health care and for trying to control costs. They do the latter by limiting expenditures, primarily through eliminating or shortening hospitalizations and by reducing reimbursements to physicians. The savings have been considerable and the profits for some of the insurance companies and HMOs have been enormous. The public is understandably concerned that the need to control medical costs will result in pressure for earlier deaths through assisted dying. Evaluation of this possibility requires answering three questions: Who is in a position to exert such pressure? Who would gain financially? and How can such a movement be recognized and avoided?

• Employers have little to gain or lose by having former employees live far into retirement. Employer contributions to benefit plans usually end with retirement, after which the plans are self-supporting. Unless the employer has a continuing responsibility for health insurance, the illness of a retiree constitutes no burden for the former employer.

• Life insurance companies have an almost unqualified interest in seeing their clients live as long as possible. Premiums have been or are being paid and income is accumulating, some to benefit the policy holder and much to benefit the insurance company. The longer this condition remains in effect, the better. As life insurance companies move into health insurance, however, their financial interests in prolonging life are significantly diluted.

• Hospitals traditionally benefited by caring for all sick patients. Provided the bills were paid, the hospital was glad to see patients stay as long as possible. From a strictly financial point of view, the hospital was also glad to see the patients go home well, so that if they got sick again they would choose the same institution. When the costs of unrestricted enterprise escalated throughout the health industry, changes were instituted. The first step the insurance/HMO industry took was to limit the amount of money hospitals could spend on their patients by establishing a payment scheme based on diagnosis-related groups (DRGs). Under that regime, an average length of hospital stay is calculated for each illness, and the hospital is reimbursed for no more than that average. Nor is the hospital allowed to charge a patient personally for the difference between the DRG-based charge and the actual costs. Numerous other mechanisms have been employed to force hospitals to cut back on their expenditures, but limiting hospitalization is the essence of most of them.

As the place where the most expensive component of health care is delivered, hospitals are caught between decreasing reimbursements from HMOs and the needs of their patients and physicians. If they should ever have to take sides, I think that they would have to side with their patients. It is in a hospital's interest to keep its beds occupied; all of the reimbursements in the world would not fill a hospital's beds if the patients decided to go elsewhere. At the same time, HMOs and insurance companies must have hospitals and must negotiate contracts that are mutually agreeable. It would be very risky for the HMOs and their participating hospitals to have contracts or agreements that include any incentive to promote assisted dying. The layers of responsibility are too complex and patient interaction too public to make hospitals reasonable conduits for cutting costs through assisted dying. Furthermore, as will be seen, better mechanisms for cost-control are available that are more compatible with the hospital's interests.

• Nursing homes have benefited from the pressure to get patients out of hospitals sooner. These institutions represent a low-cost alternative to the high cost of acute care hospitals. In that sense, too, the nursing homes profit from prolonging life when possible. Although nursing home costs per patient are related to the level of care provided, the homes might benefit from the deaths of particularly demanding patients who take up more than their share of time and effort. Nursing homes are held to strict standards by the health department, however, and any questions or complaints are usually followed up.

• Physicians also traditionally benefit from caring for patients who are sick. However ill a person may be, if his bills are paid, even in part, the physician benefits. In addition, many physicians feel a professional duty to provide some care even in the absence of reimbursement. Cost containment practices by the HMO/insurance industry have significantly reduced the incomes of many physicians, and there is public concern that if assisted dying were legal, third-party payers would put pressure on physicians to end the lives of "expensive" patients. HMOs could in theory expand their current practice of providing financial incentives for physicians to cut costs. The ambiguous role of primary physicians as gatekeepers to specialties and to more expensive care is muddied even further when primary physicians benefit by keeping the gate shut. Moderate and controlled financial incentives to physicians, with safeguards to protect patient welfare, may serve a role in containing medical costs.[27]

Expansion of this incentive system to the deliberate shortening of the lives of some patients for personal financial gain, though, would be too transparent to escape censure. The law has a responsibility to see that insurance companies and HMOs cannot provide financial incentives to physicians to shorten the lives of their patients. Even now, the public has challenged the use of "gag rules" to hide the doubtful practice of sharing the savings in health care costs with the physician, and that practice will undoubtedly be modified or dropped.

Doctors should be free to discuss any and all aspects of care, including financial, with their patients. Physicians will not be easy targets for cost cutting through assisted dying. Well-crafted guidelines, reasonable supervision, and the threat of adverse publicity, not to mention the physician's own ethical reservations, will force HMOs and insurers to seek more appropriate means for protecting their financial concerns. Far greater savings can be achieved through other mechanisms—in particular, by withdrawing or not starting treatment. It has been pointed out that the cost savings at the end of life may be too small to have any impact on the overall cost of health care.[28]

• Health insurance companies and HMOs are especially concerned with longevity and expensive illness. They collect from the healthy but pay out for the ill, so that prolonged, costly illnesses entail real losses. The industry works to recruit large numbers of young, healthy clients, to avoid older populations and those at significant risk of illness, and to absolutely refuse those who are already seriously ill. By controlling the purse, the HMO/insurance industry is in a strong position to influence hospitals and physicians and even to promote assisted dying for some patients. Although these interests could benefit from such a practice, it is not likely that they would try to do so.

For a time, the power of third-party payers to cut costs seemed to be almost unlimited and likely even to compromise the delivery of health care. But excessive cost cutting attracted public and political attention, and the pendulum is now swinging back. In one specific area—limiting new mothers to twenty-four hours of hospitalization after delivery—the outcry was loud enough to get action from Congress. The same was true for "drive-through" mastectomies, which would require outpatient surgery and no overnight hospitalization. The federal and state governments are under continuing pressure from consumers and providers to oversee the practices of the managed care industry, particularly with respect to denial of services to patients, choice of physicians, exchange of information between physicians and patients (gag rules), and loss of autonomy by physicians and patients.[29]

In spite of practices that seem domineering, arbitrary, and obscure, HMOs and insurance companies are not beyond control; they must sell themselves to the public. People buy into insurance plans and HMOs as individuals or as large groups. Physicians, singly and as groups, must also agree to participate. The desire of these plans to hide behind the small print is being thwarted by public pressure for open disclosure. Pushing for the earlier deaths of any group of patients (the demented, for example) would be scandalous for an industry that wants to avoid unfavorable publicity. The strict criteria that would have to be met, particularly in hospitals or nursing homes, would leave assisted dying open to inspection and criticism. It would be far easier to suggest restricted use of antibiotics for acute infections or to limit immediate transfer of some patients from nursing homes to hospitals, both of which strategies already fit well within the concept of DNR orders.

Real savings could come from withholding or withdrawing treatment as early in a fatal disease as reasonable rather than shortening by a few days or weeks the lives of a relatively small number of people at their own request. Both withholding and withdrawing treatment are subtle, easily accomplished without undue notice, and already commonly employed when people are fatally ill. The ethical aspects of medical futility are beginning to receive attention and will undoubtedly become more important if financial constraints tighten, because they entail much less difficult moral and political issues than do more aggressive strategies. Significantly, insurance companies and HMOs have largely avoided this controversial subject. People on dialysis or respirators cost enormous amounts of money, and there is no pressure to cut back on these supportive measures. The dangers of appearing uncaring and mercenary are too obvious to be risked, even for significant savings.

• The government is under pressure to control the cost of health care. At the same time it is expected to find some way to extend protection to as many as forty million people who have no insurance, and some observers expect these numbers may even increase.[30] Medicare, the safety net extended to all citizens over the age of sixty-five, is limited in scope and may run out of money in the coming years. Extension of medical care to the unprotected element of the population would require a major revision of priorities in the federal budget, quite possibly increased taxes as well. Failure of the recent attempt of the government to overhaul the health care system shows how complex the problem is and how many divergent interests must be taken into consideration. Financial concerns are strong and speak more loudly in this country than in many others, but other interests are also very powerful and equally vocal.

The federal government may someday have to manage the entire health care system, assuming many of the responsibilities now delegated to insurance companies and HMOs. In matters of cost containment, it will be fully answerable to the public. As tempting as it might be to cite financial pressure as a powerful force on the slippery slope, foreclosure on life, in the form of enforced or encouraged early death, is unlikely to be part of the solution of cost containment. The numbers would be far too small and the savings too meager to make an impact.

The United States is going to have a continuous political struggle to find a way to provide affordable health care for all of its citizens, but it can hardly do so at the expense of any vulnerable group, particularly the aged, when that population is going to be larger than ever and is quite capable of expressing itself. A legislator who offends any group with the size and political influence that the elderly can now wield risks an unhappy reckoning at election time.

Laws and institutions must go hand in hand with the progress of the human mind as that becomes more developed, more enlightened, as new discoveries are made, new truths discovered, and manners and opinions change with the change of circumstances. Institutions must advance also to keep pace with the times. *Thomas Jefferson*

7 The Legal Basis for Assisted Dying

Most laws concerning death and dying are made by state legislatures. Ideally, complicated issues like assisted dying should be examined by lawmakers who understand the intricacies of the problem and are willing to work on the details to create acceptable laws. But lawmakers are elected and are therefore subject to political and financial pressures from the general public and special-interest groups to such an extent that emotionally laden issues are often avoided altogether. Given the acrimony generated by some issues, it is not surprising that legislators are reluctant to reexamine and modify venerable laws that may now be outdated.[1]

The unwillingness of state legislatures to take on controversial issues led citizens in a few states, primarily in the Midwest and West, to exercise a presumably more democratic approach to legislation through public initiative. In states that recognize this prerogative, any issue that has enough public support may be voted on by the general public. This approach has its own serious shortcomings. The public at large may be less well educated or prepared to deal with complex issues than are state legislators. Moreover, the proposed law usually cannot be modified by any process of debate and negotiation but must be accepted or rejected as written. Referenda are very expensive, and the public is vulnerable to political pressure through media blitzes by well-financed interest groups. Finally, popular appeal can be emotional, and laws that originate this way are not necessarily fair or legally acceptable.

Although people accuse the judiciary of creating laws, the courts can only review existing laws and approve or disapprove them, primarily on the basis of federal or state constitutions. Still, this power is formidable. In striking down existing laws, the courts essentially force the legislatures to review and reject or modify regulations that may be inappropriate or out of date. Usually less political than legislatures, the courts are better able to address unpopular issues. In recent years, the courts have had a major impact on social progress in the form of civil and individual rights. The review process takes place in both state and federal courts. Any issue that reaches the level of a state supreme court or a federal circuit court of appeals can be further appealed to the U.S. Supreme Court, which then decides whether to review the case. Assisted dying is such an important issue that it has already been argued before the entire federal judiciary system, and it will continue to appear in the courts for many years.

The U.S. Constitution and Personal Rights

Although the United States Constitution does not define the term *right,* it was built on a foundation of intellectual and historical experience extending back over centuries of development of Western philosophy and English law.[2] Realizing that there are areas of personal concerns and privacy that should be outside of government control, the Constitution described a government with limited power over the individual. These rights were better defined in the first ten amendments, which were passed together in 1791 and became known as the Bill of Rights. Issues not specifically included in the original document have been "read into" the Constitution by its later interpreters, usually on the U.S. Supreme Court. The trend has been to extend the umbrella of individual protection provided by the Constitution. "Specific guarantees in the Bill of Rights have penumbras, formed by emanations from those guarantees that help give them life and substance."[3] As such, certain explicitly stated constitutional guarantees give rise to unstated "zones of privacy," which the government may not invade.

The Fourteenth Amendment extends the protection of the U.S. Constitution to the citizens of the individual states and declares that no state can "deprive any person of life, liberty or property without *due process* of law; nor deny any person within its jurisdiction the *equal protection* of the laws." These two clauses have been the cornerstones of the advancement of personal rights in recent years. Each state also has its own constitution. Some of these differ significantly from the U.S. Constitution, with greater emphasis on autonomy and personal rights and on protection of privacy, which is not mentioned specifically in the federal document.

Prominent throughout the evolution of Western thought has been the right to privacy, protecting personal decisions that are intimate and related to control over one's own destiny. Since its beginning, the Supreme Court has struggled with the concept of personal rights and liberty. In so doing it developed a stratification of different levels of human rights. The highest level, fundamental rights, have been described in various court decisions as "implicit in the concept of ordered liberty," such that "neither liberty nor justice would exist if they were sacrificed."[4] Fundamental rights have also been characterized as those liberties that are deeply rooted in the nation's history and tradition. These rights are so basic as to require heightened judicial protection. They may be voided by the states only for compelling state interest and then only in the narrowest and most limited sense applicable to the specific case. These are the rights reflected in the Bill of Rights and include the freedoms of assembly, speech, and worship. Through the Fifth and the Fourteenth Amendments of the Constitution, these fundamental rights have been extended to include various elements of privacy, including marriage, contraception, and abortion. These particular issues also illustrated that tradition and historical precedence are not essential prerequisites for a fundamental right, for some of them, including interracial marriage and abortion, were restricted by law and public bias for centuries. As Justice William Brennan wrote in a key opinion, "The right of personal privacy includes 'the interest in independence in making certain kinds of important decisions.' . . . Whether or not to beget or bear a child is at the very heart of this cluster of constitutionally protected choices."[5]

The next step down from a fundamental right is a "liberty interest." Although constitutionally protected by the concept of due process, a liberty interest is more vague and therefore more easily outweighed by state concerns. This category gives the states more latitude to void or limit a specific expression of personal freedom to protect its own interests. Recently the court has moved away from the concept of fundamental rights to the adoption of a continuum approach, almost a sliding scale, in which specific rights are matched against each other and against their respective state interests to establish an acceptable balance. In the only case involving termination of life examined by the Supreme Court so far, the Court considered removal of life support to be a liberty interest and not a fundamental right.[6]

State Interests

The constitutional right to privacy and liberty must be balanced against the interests of the state in preserving existing laws. The state interests that oppose physician-assisted dying include preservation of life, prevention of suicide, safeguarding the integrity of the medical profession, and protection of innocent third parties. Forty-four states have laws against assisted suicide.[7]

Probably the most basic state interest is the preservation of life, which goes beyond the life of a particular individual to upholding the sanctity of life in general. This is clearly an interest rooted in religious tradition. The essential question is what the state's interest is in keeping alive for a few extra days an old man who is suffering and near death and who wishes to die. The courts have found that the state's interest in preserving such a life is limited when it is the person's own life that is at stake and that this interest must take into consideration the medical condition and wishes of the person whose life is involved. There are already exceptions to the general goal of preserving life, in that most states now allow a patient to reject life-preserving medical measures. This can even be done by means of advance instructions, through living wills and durable powers of attorney.

The state has an interest in preventing most suicides. When circumstances may improve with help and time, every effort should be made to avoid premature and senseless loss of life. As we have seen, however, a blanket prohibition against suicide oversimplifies the problem by lumping all suicides together, rational and irrational. Like the preservation of life, this state interest decreases when the patient is suffering and dying. The decision to end suffering may be neither senseless nor premature, and laws that require unnecessary suffering can be cruel.

The religious origins of these first two state interests have little relevance for those who share different beliefs, and they have little basis in constitutional law. The Ninth Circuit Court of Appeals even questioned whether the notion of suicide was appropriate for patients electing to forgo treatment or for those requesting help in dying: "We believe that there is a strong argument that a decision by a terminally ill patient to hasten by medical means a death that is already in process, should not be classified as suicide."[8]

Some feel that new laws would not limit suicide to adults or to competent people. But the existence of a constitutional right does not prevent the state from imposing reasonable restrictions. States forbid marriage to minors, incompetents, or those with living spouses. A person judged incompetent, who cannot legally consent to any medical procedure on his own behalf, would thus be ineligible for assisted dying.

The state may feel that it has an interest in preserving traditional medical ethics. This opinion highlights a strange symbiotic relationship between the state and the medical profession, at least as represented by the American Medical Association. Each cites the other to support its own ethical or legal position. One even wonders why the integrity of the medical profession needs the protection of the law on this issue. Physicians have had to deal with death from disease far longer than the law has. Traditional medical ethics is being challenged and is already at variance with the thinking of many practicing physicians who feel that it is all right to be compassionate in the face of intense suffering. When laws against assisted dying run counter to the personal ethics and morality of the physician, acts of assistance are carried out in secret. If rules against helping people die have been sidestepped for centuries, the publicly defined role for physicians is clearly too narrow.

This mutual interdependence of the medical profession and the state to uphold traditional medical ethics and equally traditional laws is clearly unstable because either may change at any time. The medical profession and our laws are too robust to be significantly damaged by adapting to social change and embracing any single new issue, particularly when the issue is recognized as controversial, with forceful arguments on both sides. Contrary to some dire predictions, the integrity of the medical profession was not undermined by allowing patients to refuse treatment or physicians to perform abortions.

In addition to protecting families and dependent children, the state has an interest in protecting any possible innocent third parties. But concern about an unknown innocent third party should not get in the way of properly addressing the needs of the known innocent first party, namely, the patient. Sick people are guilty of nothing except being fatally ill. Few members of society exceed in vulnerability those who are dying slowly and painfully. Many now already undergo far more injury than could possibly be visited on others in the future, if protected by reasonable oversight and precautions. It should not be necessary to choose between today's known innocents and future unknown innocents. We have the moral, ethical, and intellectual ability to protect both. Physicians are not eager to dispatch their patients, and lawmakers are not eager to pass irresponsible laws. Avoiding the issue altogether for fear that future excesses cannot be prevented is neither compassionate nor responsible.

The Stepping Stones of Related Issues

Most state legislatures have been reluctant to address controversial end-of-life issues. On the other hand, the courts have provided the public and physicians a real service. In recognition of the importance of some of these problems, many of the cases were allowed to move on to higher courts even after the patients had died. The legal stepping stones that have prepared the way for consideration of assisted dying stretch back over many years. Each of them represented a challenge to existing laws passed by individual state legislatures, some so old as to have essentially been forgotten. In general, the individual cases cited reflect a strong trend toward increased individual freedom and autonomy.

The modern history of a constitutional right to privacy began with two cases concerning the use of contraceptives. In 1965 the U.S. Supreme Court ruled in *Griswold v. Connecticut* that states could not prohibit the use of contraceptives by married adults. Shortly thereafter the court extended this ruling to unmarried adults. In *Griswold,* Justice Arthur Goldberg stated that "the right to privacy is a fundamental personal right, emanating from the totality of the constitutional scheme under which we live."[9] He went on to cite a famous dissent by Justice Louis Brandeis: "The makers of our Constitution undertook to secure conditions favorable to the pursuit of happiness. They recognized the significance of man's spiritual nature, of his feelings and of his intellect. . . . They sought to protect Americans in their beliefs, their thoughts, their emotions and their sensations. They conferred, as against the government, the right to be let alone—the most comprehensive of rights and the right most valued by civilized men."[10]

The next major step in codifying the right to privacy came in 1973, when the U.S. Supreme Court extended that right to abortion in deciding *Roe v. Wade.*[11] One of the most contentious decisions that the court has ever made, Roe has been on the verge of being overturned several times since.[12] It is also one of two Supreme Court decisions that are closely related to assisted dying. As we have seen, laws prohibiting abortion were passed throughout the country in the latter half of the nineteenth century, primarily at the behest of conservative religious groups and the nascent American Medical Association.[13] The issue then lay dormant until the 1960s, when several groups began to examine it anew and recommended in 1962 that laws throughout the country be liberalized to permit abortion for the physical or mental health of the pregnant woman, if the fetus was likely to be severely defective, or if the pregnancy had resulted from rape or incest.

That same year, the country heard of the widely publicized case of an American television personality.[14] Sherri Finkbine requested an abortion of her two-month pregnancy because she had taken Thalidomide and feared that her infant would be deformed. Refused an abortion in her home state, she went to Sweden, where the procedure was legal. The fetus was indeed deformed. The publicity surrounding the case, as well as an outbreak of German measles, also known to damage the fetus, focused public attention on the inflexible laws against abortion in many states. Several states began to reconsider their laws, as did the AMA, in 1967, and by 1973 nineteen states had enacted more liberal laws on abortion.

It was against this background that the Supreme Court ruled in 1973 on *Roe v. Wade*. Roe was the fictitious name for a twenty-one-year-old divorced woman who had a five-year-old child (in the custody of Roe's mother) and who was again pregnant. With both a low income and a poor education, she was an ideal candidate to test a Texas law against abortion, dating back to the 1850s, that declared it unlawful to have or attempt an abortion for any reason except to save the life of a mother. Similar laws were in force in most other states. The Supreme Court declared these laws unconstitutional by a vote of seven to two. The most far-reaching aspect of the Court's decision was that it was based on the right to privacy. Furthermore, the majority ruled that a woman had a fundamental right to elect to have an abortion in the first trimester, a prerogative that could be voided only by a "compelling state interest."

The *Roe v. Wade* decision has come under unrelenting attack throughout the country, even in the Supreme Court itself. Various states have tried to limit a woman's access to abortion. Two cases have been critical. In *Webster v. Reproductive Health Services* the Supreme Court allowed the states to regulate abortion in the second trimester of pregnancy for purposes of protecting fetal life.[15] It also ruled that the use of public facilities for abortion could be withheld by the individual states, signifying that the constitutional right of a woman to have an abortion did not extend to economic entitlement. This ruling represented a retrenchment by the Court from its original stand on abortion and raised the question of how far it would allow the states to go. When a twelve-year Republican reign in the White House gave the Supreme Court a conservative majority, the possibility arose that *Roe v. Wade* might be reversed.

In 1992 the Supreme Court heard a second important case related to abortion, *Planned Parenthood of Southeastern Pennsylvania v. Casey.*[16] The Court upheld the state of Pennsylvania in its desire to apply several limitations on abortion, including a twenty-four-hour waiting period before an abortion could be performed and so-called informed consent, or mandatory notification of the woman about the availability of information about embryonic and fetal development. Far more important, the Casey decision downgraded a woman's prerogative to terminate an unwanted pregnancy from a fundamental right to a liberty interest, expanding the states' ability to further restrict abortions. The final decision upheld the right of women to have abortions, but only by a 5–4 majority. Writing for the majority, Justices O'Connor, Kennedy, and Souter declared: "It is a promise of the Constitution that there is a realm of personal liberty which the government may not enter. . . . At the heart of liberty is the right to define one's own concept of existence, of [the] meaning of the universe, and of the mystery of human life."[17]

Meanwhile, as the battle over privacy and autonomy was waged in the courts over abortion, a young woman's tragedy in 1975 focused the nation's attention on the issue of the right to refuse medical treatment and life support. Karen Ann Quinlan was twenty-one years old when she collapsed with respiratory failure at a party from an injudicious combination of alcohol and drugs.[18] She stabilized in a persistent vegetative state, existing on a respirator and being nourished through a tube.[19] When it was clear that she would not recover, her parents requested that the respirator be removed. Her physicians refused. In September, five months after Quinlan had gone into the coma, the trial judge backed the physician and the hospital, denying the father's request.

The case went to the New Jersey Supreme Court. A spokesman for the Catholic Church supported the father's position. The court declared that the state's interest in the preservation of life had been reduced to monitoring the patient and maintaining bodily functions and that the patient's interest, administered by her father, outweighed the interest of the physicians. Citing the right of privacy, the court stated that "the State's interest *contra* weakens and individual's right to privacy grows as the degree of bodily invasion increases and the prognosis dims. Ultimately, there comes a point when the individual's rights overcome the State interest." As a result, Quinlan was taken off the ventilator in 1976. Surprisingly, she resumed sponta neous respiration and was transferred from the hospital to a nursing home, where she was maintained on tube feedings until she died of infection in 1985. Clearly the family, who are devout Catholics and who wished to see an end to their daughter's suffering, were not willing to take the step of removing the feeding tube. It would be several years before a family or the courts would consider such an act. This was the first court decision to enunciate the constitutional right to privacy as a basis for withdrawing or withholding treatment, and the first to allow a guardian to speak for a comatose patient to that effect. The court also noted that refusal of medical intervention was not considered the same as self-inflicted deadly harm or suicide.

Because the Quinlan case was settled by the New Jersey Supreme Court, the decision was binding only in that state. In following years, however, the courts of several states examined similar cases and the body of common law was extended significantly, to include the following points:

1. Mentally retarded patients who have never been competent have the right to refuse treatment that can be expressed through a surrogate or guardian.
2. A competent adult who is terminally ill has a right to discontinue an extraordinary form of life support (a respirator, in the specific case), and such a death should be considered as having resulted from natu ral causes and not suicide or killing.
3. No significant distinction exists between extraordinary forms of life support, such as the use of a respirator or dialysis, and ordinary measures, including all forms of artificial feeding.

4. The right to refuse treatment should not be limited to those who are comatose or terminally ill but should take into consideration the quality of life as well as the quantity.

5. The substituted judgment of a spouse for a comatose person to refuse artificial feeding should be honored.[20]

The case of Nancy Cruzan ends this summary because it was the only case revolving on the right to refuse treatment that has reached the U.S. Supreme Court. Cruzan was a young woman whose car skidded on a rural road in January 1983.[21] She suffered severe brain damage that evolved into a persistent vegetative state. She required tube feedings but did not need mechanical respiration. In 1987, with no improvement, her parents asked the Missouri Rehabilitation Center to discontinue the feedings. In many respects this was similar to the Quinlan case, in which the court affirmed constitutional rights to liberty and privacy and the common-law right to preserve bodily integrity. But because there was no respiratory tube to remove, only a feeding tube, which was not considered medical treatment, the director of the center wanted to have a court order before fulfilling the family's request. He was concerned about the line between killing and allowing to die. The Missouri Supreme Court ruled that the state's interest in protecting life outweighed the patient's and parents' rights and that a parent could not decide for an incompetent child without clear evidence of what the child's desires were. The case went on to the U.S. Supreme Court, which agreed almost unanimously that everyone has the right to refuse treatment, including tube feeding. But the Court took a much narrower view in agreeing that the state of Missouri could require clear and convincing evidence of what Nancy Cruzan's own desires were and did not have to accept the petition of her parents.

This decision essentially denied federal court protection for incompetent patients unless they had been previously competent and farsighted enough to make their wishes perfectly clear well in advance. Excluded were those who had never been competent (the severely retarded), the many who had been competent previously but had never expressed their wishes (that is, had made no living will or surrogate appointment), and those whose wishes, when they were autonomous, were too vaguely expressed to be accepted by the state. Still, the ruling is not as restrictive in practice as it appears in theory. Only two states, Missouri and New York, have set standards specifically for feeding tubes and require unequivocal evidence of what the person would have wanted. Most states accept the decision of a reasonable surrogate—that is, a spouse or parent—and consider tube feeding to be similar to any other form of medical intervention. The U.S. Supreme Court eventually decided 5–4 in favor of the Missouri courts and against the parents of Nancy Cruzan. The feeding tube was left in. But the publicity brought out several people who had known her not as Cruzan but under her married name and who volunteered that when she was well, she had discussed with them her desire not ever to have to live with any form of a medical support system. This testimony was presented to the original trial judge, who accepted it and allowed the tube to be removed. Her death followed about a week later.

In their decision the Supreme Court affirmed that everyone has a right to personally refuse any form of medical treatment or support, including tube feeding. The Court agreed with Missouri, however, that the state could limit that right by refusing to accept a proxy or a surrogate. Finally, the decision classified the right to refuse treatment or life support as a liberty interest rather than a fundamental right, making it much more vulnerable to interpretation and interference by individual states.

A common theme in many of these and other similar refusal-of-treatment cases is the desire of the courts, both federal and state, to sidestep the question of suicide. The courts have been restrictive and self-protective in interpreting deaths as having been due to disease rather than self-imposed, ruling that all of the requests by competent people to remove their life support systems were to rid themselves of the machines and die from their diseases rather than to directly end their own lives. Change will require some acceptance of rational suicide, or the use of a different terminology, to apply to the seriously ill who wish to die.

The People Speak

Although the legal stepping stones show a progressively broader interpretation of individual rights and freedom with respect to defining privacy and self determination, none of them have dealt directly with assisted dying. Recognizing the reluctance of their legislatures to deal with this problem, the citizens of three states recently have tried to create their own laws through referenda. In November 1991, Washington State Initiative 119 was defeated 54 to 46 percent. A year later California Proposition 161 was voted down by the same margin.

In November 1994 the voters of Oregon were presented with ballot measure 16, the Oregon Death with Dignity Act. This was narrower and better defined than the measures that had been voted down in Washington and California. The major difference was that physician assistance was limited to assisted suicide, and euthanasia was not addressed. Oregon voters approved the act, 52–48 percent. The Oregon referendum took an unexpected turn, the legality of which was not clear, when the state legislature insisted on having a second referendum on the same question. This was held in November 1997, with the surprising result that 60 percent of the voters favored physician-assisted suicide. Some observers have suggested that the large majority resulted from voter resentment of outside pressure. It was estimated by the Hemlock Society that the Catholic Church spent four million dollars and the AMA another million in trying to influence the voters. In addition, there may also have been an element of resentment against the state legislature for infringing on the rights of the voters by not accepting the results of the original referendum.

Oregon's new law undoubtedly has more tests to withstand.

One constitutional challenge by a federal district judge was reversed by the Ninth Circuit Court of Appeals, but more will surely follow. Pressure has also been applied to the Food and Drug Administration to revoke the narcotics license of any physician in Oregon who provides prescriptions for drugs that a patient may use to end his or her life. It seems unlikely, though, that any of these diversions will undermine the new law.

The Federal Courts and Assisted Dying

In 1994 a different approach, modeled after *Roe v. Wade,* was taken to challenge the laws against assisted dying. Compassion in Dying brought a suit against the state of Washington on behalf of three patients, with advanced breast cancer, AIDS, and emphysema, respectively, and five physicians who were treating these patients.[22] All of the patients were competent and terminally ill. All wanted to end their lives with the assistance of their physicians. The five physicians were willing to provide the requested drugs if it were not prohibited under Washington law. The request was clearly for physician-assisted suicide, not for euthanasia. Judge Barbara Rothstein of the U.S. District Court of the Western District of Washington State in Seattle ruled the existing law unconstitutional. According to the judge's decision, the law placed undue burden on the exercise of the liberty interest of the Fourteenth Amendment by prohibiting physician-assisted dying; furthermore, it violated the right of equal protection under that same amendment because people who had artificial support systems could discontinue them.

The state appealed this ruling to the U.S. Court of Appeals for the Ninth Circuit.[23] After a three-judge panel reversed the opinion of Judge Rothstein, the entire court reheard the case because of its "extraordinary importance." In March 1996 this court ruled 8–3 in support of the decision of Rothstein and the district court, that the laws of Washington State against assisted dying were unconstitutional. The court based its decision on the liberty interest of the patient, citing the Casey decision on abortion: "Like the decision of whether or not to have an abortion, the decision how and when to die is one of 'the most intimate and personal choices a person may make in a lifetime,' a choice 'central to personal dignity and autonomy.' A competent terminally ill adult, having lived nearly the full measure of his life, has a strong liberty interest in choosing a dignified and humane death."[24] The court also cited the U.S. Supreme Court's opinion in *Cruzan,* upholding the due process liberty interest in terminating unwanted medical treatment: "The principle that a competent person has a constitutionally protected liberty interest in refusing unwanted medical treatment may be inferred from our prior decisions."[25] The appeals court concluded that a liberty interest that includes refusal of life-sustaining treatment should also include hastening one's own death. It insisted that the liberty interest in choosing the time and manner of death includes refusing treatment and is therefore broader than "suicide."

Having determined that a person does indeed have a liberty interest in controlling the time and manner of death, the court went on to declare that the state's interest in preserving life and in preventing suicide varies from case to case. The court pointed out the need to balance a constitutionally protected interest against the state's opposing interests, noting that the liberty interest is at its peak in the case of the terminally ill, at which time the state interests are at a low point. "Not only is the state's interest in preventing such individuals from hastening their deaths of comparatively little weight, but its insistence on frustrating their wishes seems cruel indeed."[26] The court felt that abusive coercion of a person was unlikely at the terminal stages of disease and that a complete prohibition of assisted suicide was excessively restrictive in light of the many safeguards that could be provided. The circuit court of appeals declined to make an opinion on the basis of equal protection, feeling that a single constitutional violation was enough to support the judgment that it had reached.

Proponents of assisted dying used the same approach in New

York State.[27] Again, three patients requested assistance in dying. Three physicians, including Timothy Quill, after whom the case is named, submitted that they would help these patients to die, if it were legal, by providing them with prescriptions for appropriate drugs. After a district judge ruled against them, the case was appealed and was heard by the three-judge Court of Appeals for the Second Circuit. That panel reversed the district court ruling and declared unanimously that the laws of New York State forbidding physician-assisted dying were unconstitutional, but on different grounds from the Ninth Circuit Court of Washington.

The New York court felt that the right to assisted suicide did not qualify as a fundamental liberty under the due process clause of the Fourteenth Amendment, noting that the Supreme Court had been reluctant to expand its definition of fundamental rights. The court of appeals did agree, however, that the physician and patient plaintiffs were denied equal protection under existing laws, also part of the Fourteenth Amendment. This clause "requires the states to treat in a similar manner all individuals who are similarly situated." Because people in New York State who are on artificial support systems have a right to request that their treatment be discontinued, knowing that this will result in death, the court ruled, those without such support systems but suffering similar distress should have the same mortal option. Critics of this decision on the basis of equal protection claim that it fails to recognize an ethical difference between allowing a person to die and helping a person to die. But this ethical distinction is tenuous at best when one acknowledges that the patient who asks to have life-sustaining treatment discontinued knows that the result will be his death. Circuit Court Judge Calabresi concurred with the result but thought that there was also a constitutionally protected liberty interest in an individual's decision to terminate life. He pointed out that many laws of this kind are more than a century old and urged the New York State Legislature to review its statute against assisted dying that dates back to 1881 and to provide the courts with clear guidance as to what the current thinking of the public really is: "No court need or ought to make ultimate and immensely difficult constitutional decisions unless it knows that the state's elected representatives and executives—having been made to go, as it were, before the people—assert through their actions (not their inactions) that they really want and are prepared to defend laws that are constitutionally suspect."[28]

As the public concept of liberty continues to expand, the court system, and particularly the U.S. Supreme Court, have acknowledged uncertainty about where constitutionally protected liberty ends. As Justice Brennan has written, "The outer limits of this aspect of privacy have not been marked by the Court."[29] Moreover, the Supreme Court has encountered liberty interests that it would not accept, as when it ruled that homosexual conduct between consenting adults was not protected by the Constitution as a fundamental liberty. In dissenting, Justice Harry Blackmun pointed out that the majority viewed the issue much too narrowly: "This case is not about 'a fundamental right to engage in homosexual sodomy,' as the Court purports to declare. Rather, this case is about 'the most comprehensive of rights and the right most valued by civilized men,' namely, 'the right to be let alone.'"[30] The result of the decision is a patchwork arrangement of states that legally tolerate certain sexual relationships and those that prohibit them.

The Supreme Court's decision on *Cruzan* had almost the same effect. In addressing a very narrow issue, the state's right to require strong evidence of what Nancy herself would have wanted rather than accepting the petition of her parents, the Court pushed the public in the opposite direction. All but two states now accept the proxy of a close relative. Moreover, public fear of loss of personal control led Congress to pass the Self-Determination Act of 1990. A vast majority of the public favored advance directives, but in practice relatively few had taken the necessary steps. The bill required that all institutions receiving Medicare or Medicaid funding inform patients about their rights to use advance directives and to encourage them to do so. Because this bill was initially opposed by the

Catholic Church and other right-to-life groups, Congress was sub
jected to all the pressure associated with an emotional issue. The
same groups, though, have generally found the law acceptable and
even useful.[31]

The U.S. Supreme Court Decision

On January 8, 1997, the Supreme Court heard two cases involving
physician-assisted suicide, *Washington v. Glucksberg* and *Quill v.
Vacco*. In both cases the issue was whether state laws forbidding
physicians from helping certain patients to die were constitutional.
The states of Washington and New York were appealing decisions
of their respective courts of appeal. On June 26, 1997, the Court decided unanimously that the existing laws in both states did not violate the U.S. Constitution, overturning the decisions of the two circuit courts of appeal.[32]

Chief Justice William Rehnquist wrote for the Court that its
due process analysis rested on two premises: that fundamental rights
and liberties are "deeply rooted in this Nation's history and tradition" and that a careful description of the asserted fundamental liberty interest is required. "The history of the law's treatment of assisted suicide in this country," Rehnquist wrote, "has been and
continues to be one of the rejection of nearly all efforts to permit it.
That being the case, our decisions lead us to conclude that the asserted 'right' to assistance in committing suicide is not a fundamental liberty interest protected by the Due Process Clause." He went
on to state that Washington State's ban on assisted suicide was rationally related to legitimate government interests, including the
preservation of human life, prevention of suicide, protecting the integrity of the medical profession, protecting vulnerable groups, and
avoidance of a path toward voluntary euthanasia. It should be noted
that although the Supreme Court prefers to apply the due process
clause to fundamental rights and liberties that are deeply rooted in
our history and tradition, it has not always done so. Its rulings on in-

terracial marriage, suicide, birth control, and abortion all reversed laws deeply rooted and traditional in our legal thinking.

In reversing the opinion of the Second Circuit Court of Appeals for New York, Rehnquist declared that New York State's ban on assisted suicide did not treat different groups of people differently, because "*everyone,* regardless of physical condition, is entitled to refuse unwanted lifesaving medical treatment, and *no one* is permitted to assist a suicide." He went on to state that "unlike the Court of Appeals, we think the distinction between assisting suicide and withdrawing life-sustaining treatment, a distinction widely recognized and endorsed in the medical profession and in our legal traditions, is both important and logical; it is certainly rational."

These opinions were not surprising, and Rehnquist himself outlined the background for them: "We have always been reluctant to expand the concept of substantive due process because guideposts for responsible decisionmaking in the uncharted area are scarce and open-ended," and "the outlines of the 'liberty' specially protected by the Fourteenth Amendment—never fully clarified, to be sure, and perhaps not capable of being fully clarified—have at least been carefully refined by concrete examples involving fundamental rights found to be deeply rooted in our legal tradition." The current court has been very resistant to any expansion of due process or equal protection aspects of the Fourteenth Amendment.

This seemingly total rejection of physician-assisted dying by the Supreme Court was softened by several other statements on the same cases.[33] Rehnquist concluded his remarks by saying that "throughout the Nation, Americans are engaged in earnest and profound debate about the morality, legality and practicality of physician-assisted suicide. Our holding permits this debate to continue, as it should in a democratic society."

Justice David Souter, in another opinion on the same case, noted that a Supreme Court decision in favor of assisted dying at this time would be premature and would bypass experimentation and legislative judgments at the state level: "The Court should accordingly stay its hand to allow reasonable legislative consideration. While I do not decide for all time that respondents' claim should not be recognized, I acknowledge the legislative institutional competence as the better one to deal with that claim at this time."

Justice Sandra Day O'Connor emphasized the use of the double effect: "A patient who is suffering from a terminal illness and who is experiencing great pain has no legal barriers to obtaining medication, from qualified physicians, to alleviate that suffering, even to the point of causing unconsciousness and hastening death." She went on to state that "there is no reason to think the democratic process will not strike the proper balance between the interests of terminally ill, mentally competent individuals who would seek to end their suffering and the State's interests in protecting those who might seek to end life mistakenly or under pressure. States are presently undertaking extensive and serious evaluation of physician-assisted suicide and other related issues. In such circumstances, the . . . challenging task of crafting appropriate procedures for safeguarding . . . liberty interests is entrusted to the 'laboratory' of the States."

Justice Stephen Breyer stated, "The Court describes it as a 'right to commit suicide with another's assistance.' But I would [consider] a different formulation, for which our legal tradition may provide greater support. That formulation would use words roughly like a 'right to die with dignity.' But irrespective of the exact words used, at its core would lie personal control over the manner of death, professional medical assistance, and the avoidance of unnecessary and severe physical suffering combined. . . . I do not believe, however, that this Court need or now should decide whether or not such a right is 'fundamental.'"

Justice John Paul Stevens noted that there is "significant tension between the traditional view of the physician's role and the actual practice in a growing number of cases. Although as the Court concludes today, these *potential* harms are sufficient to support the State's general public policy against assisted suicide, they will not always outweigh the individual liberty interest of a particular patient. I would not foreclose the possibility that an individual plaintiff seeking to hasten her death, or a doctor whose assistance was sought, could prevail in a more particularized challenge. Future cases will determine whether such a challenge may succeed."

These modifying statements make it clear that the Supreme Court does not wish to dismiss the issue of assisted dying altogether but is inviting the states to look at it individually through their legislatures and other forums. The justices' opinions suggest that it was premature to bring this issue to the Supreme Court and that it should now be submitted to additional review by the general public, by individual states, and by the lower courts. Their statements also raise the possibility that the Supreme Court may someday review the issue again. This leaves the door ajar for the states, and for individuals and their physicians, to consider and act on their own attitudes toward assisted dying.

New Laws

The decision by the Supreme Court, overruling the opinions of two circuit courts of appeal, means that the current court finds no right to physician-assisted dying that is protected by the U.S. Constitution. This does not mean that the Court forbids assisted dying or, indeed, necessarily holds that it should be against the law. The ruling allows any state to pass laws that permit assisted dying under any applicable legal banner, including declaration of a personal right. It should be noted that the constitutions of many states differ from the U.S. Constitution in defining personal rights and privacy. It would require a separate and much more limiting action for the U.S. Supreme Court to say that the passage of a state law permitting assisted dying was too dangerous for the public to be allowed to stand. The Court has not said this. Instead, it has allowed the more liberal states to move ahead and develop legal guidelines for assisted dying, much as Oregon is doing. At the same time their ruling does not force conservative states to accept something that many citizens of those states abhor and may never willingly accept.

In the United States we have an unusual opportunity to evaluate different approaches to controversial issues like assisted dying. Experiments in only one or two states within our own borders will relieve people on both sides of the issue of the temptation to rely on the Dutch experience, developed in a society that differs significantly from our own. With the flexibility to contrast a variety of approaches, it will be possible to look closely at many aspects of assisted dying. Ultimately, we should be able to craft laws that will protect the rights of those who wish to die comfortably, with assistance, while safeguarding those who express no such interest. Laws that permit assisted dying can be repealed if they fail to protect the innocent, and other states can back away on the basis of the experience of states that have tried it.

Attempts to pass laws permitting assisted dying on a state-by-state basis will allow those who oppose it to focus their considerable national resources on each state, one at a time, as the issue comes up. Some conservative groups are disproportionately outspoken and influential. They can create confusion in public referenda and political pressure in state legislatures. Many religious organizations have abandoned a sanctity-of-life approach because of its limited appeal, and rely instead on the prediction that abuse will be impossible to control and will inevitably lead to a slippery slope of moral disintegration. It will now be possible to settle this dispute within our own culture to the extent that people want to settle it. Some, however, will oppose any attempt by any state to critically examine physician-assisted dying on a trial basis precisely because their fallback argument may be abolished by just such an experiment. They would prefer to keep the conflict alive than to have an answer.

As various states conduct their experiments, other objections will be raised: not enough time has elapsed, too much is being done behind closed doors, the data are incomplete, and so on. The opposition will also fight the issue in the courts. This was already attempted with the Lee case in Oregon.[34] The attitude of the Supreme Court will be further defined in the process. If it feels that the concept of assisted dying should be tested in the individual states, it will refuse to hear appeals or decide against them, in order to indicate that the Court is not taking issue with the basic morality or legality of assisted dying, at least at a constitutional level. As each state resolves the issue in its own way, there may eventually be pressure to consolidate their differing views. A citizen may be discriminated against simply because he lives in a conservative state. Those who are mortally ill may not find it feasible to travel to other states where assistance is available, and no state is likely to want to become the last refuge for people seeking death. At that point, the Supreme Court may step back in to mandate more uniform laws, much as it did with racial segregation. It will undoubtedly be a different court and will have available to it a background of experience and information developed in our own country.

Old Laws or No Laws

For the next few years most states are going to continue to have laws forbidding assisted dying. The differences of opinion between two important circuit courts of appeal and that of the U.S. Supreme Court, however, reflect the wide range of views within the country and the fact that the issue is far from decided. As it stands now, not only are states free to do what they want, but to a lesser degree, so are patients and their physicians.

Where does this leave people who want assisted dying and physicians who would consider helping them, even though providing such help is illegal? If the issue of assisted dying has not been settled in any way at a legal level, it has certainly not been settled at a personal one. With our courts seriously split, it is not unreasonable to think that physician-assisted dying may be wrong for some doctors and their patients, but not for others, perhaps depending on the circumstances. Moreover, even if it is wrong for everyone, it doesn't appear to be very wrong, for penalties are minimal or nonexistent. This leads one to conclude that assisted dying may be permissible in practice but not in law. Laws that cannot or are not enforced take on the character of no law at all.

We have two ways of looking at laws that are not universally accepted or obeyed.[35] The first is to recognize that our legal system is complex and stratified, with some laws that are widely accepted and binding on all, with serious sanctions for violations. Laws against murder fall into this category. Within the same legal system, however, are laws of much lesser importance, laws that carry milder sanctions or none at all, which may not even be enforced. Automobile speed limits vary from state to state and may be changed at any time. Under the best of circumstances they are not strictly or uniformly enforced. Our legal system must accommodate change, accepting a wide range of behaviors, demands, and even contradictions. One way to give the system enough flexibility to function properly, if not always fairly, is to recognize a difference between "hard laws" and "soft laws," in which the seriousness of the crime is roughly measured by the penalty exacted for infractions. Physician-assisted dying falls into the category of soft law, if only because it has never been successfully upheld when the circumstances of assistance were reasonable. On the other hand, it carries the threat of prosecution as hard law—at least manslaughter, perhaps even murder—a threat that must be taken into consideration by the physician. Soft laws, in the sense that I have applied the term to assisted dying, are tolerated precisely because our society has groups that espouse conflicting views and cannot yet reach a consensus on an issue that eventually must be resolved.

Another way of looking at laws that are not universally accepted is to recognize a legal double standard, with laws that apply to some but not others.[36] Here the law is acknowledged publicly but circumvented deliberately by those who feel justified in doing so. The few who break the law do so privately and secretly, not only to avoid detection but to allow the myth of the formal law to be protected. One example is the public official who, perhaps short of lying, dissembles and misleads Congress "for the good of the country" or "for reasons of national security." Under this system, the physician who helps a person to die would do so quietly and privately, as has often been the practice in the past. The very fact of being a physician may provide an elite status that is not extended to others. The AMA undoubtedly harbors many members who have helped people to die but protects its oppositional stand by strenuously objecting to the legalization of assisted dying. Permitting exceptions provides the law with some scope to adjust to larger social issues. It allows for latitude to meet specific needs that formal law has not accepted. It also preserves an important portal for changes in the law. Thus rapid social change, as brought about by advances in technology, tends to minimize the relevance of historical precedence and forces smaller groups, such as states or even individuals, to make their own choices. This will increasingly be the case as more patients and physicians discuss assisted dying.

A step beyond allowing some physicians to break the law secretly would be to formalize an amnesty system, such as is currently in place in the Netherlands.[37] Although physician-assisted dying would be illegal, the law could be changed to allow the prosecuting attorney to make it clear publicly that physicians who help patients to die would be legally excused and would not be prosecuted if they did so openly and within certain guidelines. It would be up to the physician to demonstrate that he or she had met the legal requirements, and failure to do so would make the whole act a punishable offense. Some physicians would welcome such a window of legal acceptance. This approach, however, would require that the physician acknowledge participating in an act that was technically illegal, which she could have performed in total secrecy, with little chance of being found out or convicted of any crime. In our litigious society, where prosecutors are elected officials with public duties to perform, the risks of this legislative compromise would probably seem too great for many physicians. They might prefer to help their patients die in secret if they could not do so under the protection of law.

It is also possible that patients might bypass their physicians altogether. With adequate information available concerning specific drugs, the enterprising patient or family might find other avenues to peaceful death. Although barbiturates are no longer the staple of sedation that they once were, they are still available through street-corner merchants. If the need becomes sufficiently great and the laws remain restrictive, a black market could evolve for the small but desperate population searching for a one-time-only opportunity to obtain drugs outside of legal channels. Indeed, a route already exists for people who are willing and able to travel outside the United States, primarily to Mexico.

Finally, absence of laws that permit and regulate assisted dying may establish the practice permanently in the privacy of the physician-patient relationship, where it began. This may not be a bad outcome, remote as it now seems. Exerting control over one's death, even with help, is a personal matter and should be recognized and accepted as such. When appropriate and requested, physician assistance may someday become a normal recognized aspect of compassionate care. Until then, the public is going to want to supervise and regulate it as well as possible. But before society can expect to have any control over assisted dying, it will first have to legalize it.

People are going to go on seeking a terminus at the end of life, whether the Church or the politicians like it or not. The doctor should be involved in making these terminations clean and safe. If the body is a dwelling, the human soul and mind deserve a dignified release from that house when it is beyond repair. . . . Responsible physicians should join forces with the public to write a new chapter in medical education that places care in death in its proper context. It is tricky. It is dangerous. But we need it and people are ready for it. It will relieve more suffering than did the discovery of anesthesia 150 years ago. *Francis D. Moore*

8
From Patients to Physicians and Policy

Throughout this book I have emphasized why I think laws permitting assisted dying are desirable. In this concluding chapter I will explain why I think that passage of such laws is inevitable and what can be done to speed up the process. I will also speak with two voices, that of a person who would like to have some control over how my life ends, including the possibility of assisted dying, and that of a physician who could be asked to provide such assistance. Being neither a legal scholar nor a public policy expert, I can only touch on these areas in very general terms. But as a surgeon who treats people with cancer, I hear what they have to say, and I know what I would like to see accomplished by changes in the law.

The inevitability of laws that permit assisted dying arises from the many inexorable changes that are taking place in our society and in its medical needs. The elderly make up the most rapidly growing segment of our population, and with advanced age comes an accumulation of illnesses that collectively can greatly weaken the body and mind. Loss of personal control and the financial distress associated with prolonged terminal illness are genuine fears. The penalties for outliving one's good health can be devastating.

Painful deaths can affect several generations. More young people see their parents and grandparents live out their final years in nursing homes, some suffering significantly from their illnesses. The trauma of witnessing a bad death leaves its own lasting impression; "I will never let that happen to me" is a common sentiment. AIDS, a newcomer to our medical and social scene, is responsible for some of the most tragic and ugly deaths that can be experienced. In searching for answers, many AIDS patients have already arrived at physician-assisted dying as the most humane way to avoid unnecessary and futile suffering. Until a "comfortable" death with a minimum of suffering becomes a right for all, the risk of having a prolonged, humiliating, and disheartening end to life hangs over every one of us, regardless of age. There is ample reason for the fears that are now being expressed by so many people.

Much has been said about the dramatic expansion of medical treatment and technology that have made it possible to cure many diseases that once were fatal at an early age. The result is that the vast benefits of modern medicine carry a significant price tag at the end of life. Long, productive lives often end in slow, uncomfortable deaths. This is no minor trend; it is a fact with which many of us may have to contend. Moreover, this expansion of technology is in midstride; any long-range planning for medical care must anticipate further major advances. Neither the public nor the medical profession wants to see a halt or even a slowdown in research that may control disease and prolong life. As individuals and as a society, we are more than willing to take our chances on what tomorrow will provide. But now we are also on the threshold of having some control, the capacity to prevent tomorrow from bringing unwanted misery. Already a significant majority thinks that doctors should be legally allowed to help some people die under at least some circumstances. This pressure for greater patient autonomy is certain to continue to build.

The past fifty years have also brought enormous changes in our moral attitudes, and even in the religious beliefs from which they were derived. Sex and reproduction have been the major areas of concern. Predictably, the popular divisions over these sensitive issues are being extended to assisted dying, with the same acrimonious debate and much of the same inflammatory language. There is an answer to this impasse, though—an answer that I think is also inevitable. Our country, indeed the entire world, is becoming more complex, with more competing ideas and ideologies and vastly more individual desires and needs to be accommodated. The result is that, in spite of ourselves, we are becoming more tolerant and accepting of others. As we strive for greater personal autonomy, we are forced to recognize and accept similar desires in others.

Physician-assisted dying is going to test the tolerance of individuals in the United States and much of the Western world as has no other personal issue. Some opponents have tried to muzzle all discussion on the basis of absolute morality. They hope to discourage any intelligent and reasonable consideration of the issue on its own merits that might lead to a closer look at the true morality in question.[1] Others argue that "even if euthanasia is legalized in some jurisdictions, physicians should refuse to participate in it and professional organizations should censure any of their members who [do]."[2] A thoughtful public should not tolerate such attitudes. In a diverse society, no group, religious or professional, should expect to force its restrictions onto everyone else. The trend is toward greater tolerance with respect to many social issues, including assisted dying, and those who suffer, and those who must watch others suffer, have every reason to expect and even demand it.

Advancing Your Own Interests

The interactions of medicine and society do not change by themselves. But they do respond to pressure, and now is the time to speak openly about assisted dying. Our inability to prevent death does not mean that we cannot have any control over it—in fact, we live in an age when we know that we can.

The cascade of pressure begins with the public—with individual patients and their families. From there it extends to their physicians and on to the medical profession, eventually reaching the lawmakers and the courts. As a patient or potential patient (and we are all potential patients), you should initiate conversations with your physician about end-of-life issues, personally confronting and forcing her to confront a subject that may be uncomfortable for both parties. Many people, knowing that a request for help in dying may challenge the religious, personal, and professional beliefs of their doctors, never bring the subject up. Although a physician may dismiss such requests with the disclaimer that such an act is against the law and therefore impossible, sympathetic doctors in increasing numbers are promising and giving their patients the help they ask for.

As requests for assisted dying become more common, physicians will be forced to choose whether or not to help. In the past, many physicians took a paternalistic stance toward the notion of patient autonomy, but patients and physicians are now being buffeted by changes in the health care system. As a result, doctors are in need of alliances that are meaningful and durable, the oldest and most honored of which is the contract with the patient. This is an opportune time for people to put pressure on their physicians for help at the end of life. Physicians should be challenged with hard questions from the one source they cannot easily ignore, their patients. While the medical profession may object institutionally to physician-assisted dying, many of the doctors who make up that profession do not. A few simple questions will determine where your doctor stands, and a few more may even influence her thinking.

A change in health plans forced me to find a primary care physician, the first such doctor to enter my adult life. After responding to many questions and undergoing a thorough exam, I asked my own question. "Suppose that ten years from now I developed cancer of the pancreas that could not be cured and was very painful. If I asked you for a prescription for Seconal that I could have on hand to end my own life if the suffering became unbearable, would you give it to me?" He said "I have, and I would." My wife's new physician responded to a similar question with almost the same words. Help may already be available.

Most of the moral debate about end-of-life medical decisions has emphasized society and the physician, with very little attention to the patient. The clear-cut intent of a patient to see his life end is overshadowed by the desire to give the physician moral protection under the umbrella of the double effect, passive euthanasia, and so on. Our courts do the same thing, trying desperately to avoid having a person who elects to discontinue life support seem responsible for his own death. But patients are moral individuals too, with needs and rights of their own, and forcing a slow and unnecessarily painful death on another is unambiguously immoral. As it is, we live under many layers of paternalism, beginning with the family and extending to our teachers, doctors, the church, and the state. Each authority professes to know what is best for us. Paternalism is absolute when we are children, but its grip weakens as we grow older and more independent. By the time we must face the end of life, most people have outgrown or bypassed some of the layers of paternalism and may be in conflict with others. Overcoming this paternalism requires a strong sense of autonomy and willingness to assert it. In dealing with the medical profession, people must ask for what they want. Legalized assisted dying will arrive sooner if people push for it, and the physician's office is the place to begin. But the right will not be simply handed over. It will have to be convincingly argued for by those who stand to gain (or lose) the most—patients and the public.

End-of-life concerns should be focused on the patient rather than on the physician or the law.[3] Agony from advanced disease that is severe enough to make a person wish to have his life end is the same agony regardless of the mode of death, be it refusal of treatment, the double effect of drugs, suicide, assisted suicide, or euthanasia. The underlying reason that the patient wants earlier death is to end his suffering. Concerns of physicians and the law should be secondary. Physicians should be as supportive as possible, regardless of what is required, at a point in life when the patient's needs are greater than ever, even if only for short time. The laws that are imposed should be broad and general, leaving most decision making to patients and their physicians, with as little oversight as possible. As physicians and the law increasingly respect the rights of patients, the need for excuses to rationalize the intent to die or to assist in death will be reduced.

Autonomy also has limits that should be understood. Suicide, which is legal, is a private act. Because it requires no interaction with anyone else, it is also the only completely autonomous step that one can take to end his life. As soon as a physician is included to assist in any way, autonomy must be shared. The patient shares autonomy in finding a physician who is willing to help and in agreeing on terms, the timing, and the method to be used. Regardless of whether assisted dying is legal or not, some negotiation with the physician will be necessary, and some compromise should be expected. She is not obliged to accept the responsibility, and she is free to set her own requirements. Finally, legalization of assisted dying will introduce specific requirements, including some form of public oversight. The confidential nature of the patient-physician relationship will necessarily be qualified. This invasion of the privacy of both patient and physician is the unavoidable cost of legal approval and protection.

Some would actually deny you your autonomy altogether, on the grounds that much of your "condition"—the severity of your suffering, your life expectancy, your competence, the voluntariness of your request, the nature of your terminal illness, and even the essence of your personality—cannot be measured.[4] But many aspects of life vary widely from one individual to another and defy accurate measurement, including most of the qualities that make us individuals, with reasoning and reasons of our own. The meaning of life is a totally personal and private matter, frequently defying definition, no less measurement. The vagaries and imprecision of life are factors that must be accepted in every important decision that we make, including the decision to request or provide assisted dying. You have every reason to be in control. It is your life, your death, and it should be your right to make your own evaluation and decision.

You also have good reason to question the state's real interest in preserving for a few extra days the life of a person who is dying. It seems pale when used as an excuse to require unnecessary suffering. Some would say that the state must be concerned about the possibility of injury to others, even if doing do so directly metes out very real injury to those requesting relief. But as more people experience or witness actual injury, they are becoming skeptical of concerns about possible injury to unknown persons in the vague future. It seems inappropriate to continue to cause deliberate harm out of fear that we may some day stumble helplessly into a different harm, one that is hypothetical and can be avoided by instituting appropriate safeguards.

You can arouse a lot of sympathy for the cause of assisted dying by sharing your concerns with friends, support groups, religious and community groups, doctors and other health care providers, newspapers, and even the local medical society. Everyone thinks that he is the only one who wants compassionate discussion and even help at the end of life. Nothing can be further from the truth. Many people share the same concern and they can gain strength in precisely that way—by *sharing* the concern. Support groups provide excellent opportunities to exchange information and can become sounding boards for dissatisfaction with medical care, even near the end of life. These groups can even exploit the medical community's interest in avoiding scandals, for severe suffering can be truly scandalous. Public disclosure creates pressure and change, often quite rapidly. The Quinlan case was perceived as a scandal, and it altered society's concept of the needs of the individual at the end of life.

Beyond putting pressure on physicians, you can take the issue

to members of your state legislatures. Had the U S Supreme Court
upheld the opinions of the appeals courts, every state would already
have had to examine and modify its laws against assisted dying. As
it is, the Court's ruling allows any state to change its laws, but none
must do so. The result is that legalization of assisted dying will be a
prolonged and piecemeal process. It will be nudged ahead by pres
sure from the public, as it was in Oregon, but the route will be selected with extreme caution and at first the pace will be slow. As experience accumulates and personal suffering and frustration spark
public awareness, momentum will increase. The desire for personal
control at the end of life and the simple logic of avoiding unnecessary suffering are two imperatives that will be impossible to sidestep
indefinitely.

The Physician in the Middle

Until laws prohibiting assisted dying are changed, physicians are going to be in a very difficult position, caught between the needs of
their patients and legal proscriptions imposed by the states. In won-
dering why physicians would help their patients to die, knowing that
it is against the law, we have only to look back a few years to the
medical acceptance of abortion, when it, too, was illegal. I lived
through that era. Some physicians did many abortions, undoubtedly
for money. Most abortions, however, were performed by qualified
gynecologists for more altruistic reasons. Friendship sometimes
played a role: physicians could usually find colleagues who would
"help out." Understanding and compassion for a woman's distress
were common motives, as were respect for autonomy and the right
of the woman to decide for herself. The balance was increasingly
weighted in favor of overlooking laws that no longer seemed valid.
All of these reasons appear to be applicable to assisted dying today.

New laws should protect both patients and their physicians. I
have detailed proposed guidelines elsewhere. My main concern is
that the requirements not be made so complicated and elaborate

that they exclude most people. Pain and suffering should not be subjected to formal evaluation. It should be enough for the physician to confirm that the patient has a fatal disease that is causing appreciable suffering. Beyond that, evaluation of the suffering is strictly a subjective one that must be left to the patient.

A major purpose of any law that permits assisted dying is to provide authorization and protection for the physician. If the death was appropriate for the patient's medical condition, and the legal requirements met, the physician should be free of any liability whatsoever. A physician who participates in assisted dying would need protection from family members who were not involved in the decision and from outside individuals or groups who object to assisted dying in principle. Although patient and physician may agree between themselves on assisted death, the formality of their contract could be hard to prove at a later date. Today's video technology can provide inexpensive and convincing evidence of the discussions that take place between physician, patient, and family and the steps that are agreed upon.

It has been seriously suggested that our current laws against assisted dying be maintained but physicians be permitted and almost encouraged to help appropriate patients die, if they are willing to accept the risks. Supporters of this point of view feel that assisted dying is occasionally morally acceptable but that it should not be legalized. As one medical oncologist/ethicist put it, "By establishing a social policy that keeps physician assisted suicide and euthanasia illegal, but recognizes exceptions, we would adopt the correct moral view . . . . Such a policy would recognize that ending a life by physician assisted suicide or euthanasia is an extraordinary and grave event."[5] Similarly, it was reported that some panelists on the New York State Task Force on Life and Law held that "assisted suicide might be appropriate for some incurable individuals suffering from intractable pain," but the panelists "prefer that such patients get help quietly from thoughtful and courageous doctors willing to violate the law."[6]

This ambivalence may reflect the doubts of some about the system or the universe of doctors to be adequately selective or careful. An oncologist and ethicist in my hospital put it this way: "To legalize assisted dying would create a license for an act which I think should only be participated in by very few physicians and then only after serious reflection. The current law proscribes the deed but looks with mercy upon its performance. There are boundaries one should not overstep save with very real deliberation." But there is no reason why willingness to assist in dying would be confined to particularly good or careful physicians outside the law anymore than it would be if the entire process were legalized.

In addition to burdening physicians with a legal risk that many would find unacceptable, such a system would also provide no guidelines for the physician in terms of patient eligibility, methods of helping at the time of death, and so on. We may have a tendency to confuse legal risk to the physician with guidelines, although they are quite separate entities. Guidelines have already evolved, but physicians do not necessarily have reason to follow them. Indeed, there would be no way of knowing whether a physician who assisted in a death followed any guidelines at all. Written requests and witnesses would be optional, and second opinions would be out of the question. Similarly, without laws that permit physician-assisted dying, the public will have no possibility of overseeing the practice. With no guaranteed protection whatsoever for the physician, this would be an unstable and therefore temporary compromise.

If You Want Help

Most of this book has necessarily taken a somewhat distanced, theoretical approach to the question of assisted dying. Now we shall examine the steps you may someday wish to take and some of the conflicts you can expect in asking for assistance.

The first step in considering the possibility of physician-assisted dying is to examine or develop a personal philosophy concerning the end of your life. Some people go into every experimental trial available and fight to the end, with little thought of what the end may be like. Others can see at least the possibility that the loss of quality of life may tip the balance and that they will wish to have the option of an earlier death. Finally, there is a group of people who on principle want to have greater control, to be able to pick the time and place of exit. Without at all being defeatists, they accept impending death and want to be in control.

Asking for assistance requires acceptance that you are indeed dying and that planning it may be personally preferable to letting it just happen. Many people never reach that point, being buoyed by hope or deterred by denial, and others reach such a level of acceptance too late to go through the formalities required to obtain help. Still others, for personal or religious reasons, are content or even glad to accept whatever comes. A few, however, wish to have some control over the time and circumstances of death, even to the point of asking for assistance from a physician. Full acceptance provides an opportunity to go beyond passive resignation to active planning and a voluntary confrontation with death, seen by many as the ultimate exercise in autonomy. If this is your approach, you may find dying at home appealing, at least in theory, for it provides much greater freedom to exercise your will.

The decision to die, with or without help, is exceedingly difficult, with many questions to examine and conflicts to resolve. Small wonder, then, that people in this situation are ambivalent and need psychological room to maneuver. Concern about advancing the time of one's death, even by just a few days, is understandable and should be accepted as part of the necessary process of rationalization, weighing good against bad. It is not a sign of emotional instability but rather recognition of the enormity of the step being contemplated. Two strong forces are at work: the desire for relief from suffering and the will to live.

Some feel that ambivalence in the face of such a choice is a sign of indecisiveness and that assistance in dying should not be offered to someone who is so uncertain. But just because a choice for earlier death over longer life is difficult is no reason to deny a person the right to make such a choice.[7] People sometimes compartmentalize their dying, cutting it off from the rest of their being. One patient I knew was a girl in her teens. On one hand she would talk about going to college in September and wonder where she should apply. Five minutes later she would talk about the realization that she didn't have much time left. Total commitment to dying is too much to ask anyone who has ever enjoyed life; I would question the values of a person who found the decision to end life easy.

THE DOCTOR'S ROLE

Our doctors need to know what our own thoughts are, and we should not hesitate to tell them.[8] As more people insist not only on maximum comfort but on the right to shorten life if they wish, more physicians will become comfortable with the idea of providing the necessary help. You should ask for what you want, and do so when you are well, or as early as possible in your illness. Indeed, you should push your doctor for a promise to provide help if it is ever needed. Late in illness, your options may be limited to the point where someone else may have to take control and act on your behalf. There is no reason why at some time earlier in the disease you should not be able to speak and even act on your own behalf. All the important people should be present: you, who are suffering and dying; your family, who are experiencing it with you; and the physician who has the knowledge and the means to fulfill your request. You should take the opportunity to make your wishes known while your ability to make a clear-headed decision is indisputable.

The presence of your physician at the time of death could provide enormous moral support. With her knowledge of the drugs available, she could assure you that the act will not fail. In sharing in the planning and offering to be present at the time of death, she also opens the door to close family members and others who are close to you. If she is willing to be there, others may be too. The physician must be able to enter into such an agreement voluntarily. If for any reason she is unwilling to help with death, she should tell you immediately. Once having agreed to help, she is honor-bound to do so. If it is clear that your physician will not consider providing any help or will not even discuss the subject with you, you may find it desirable to seek out another who is more understanding. This, too, will become more common as attitudes change.

FAMILY

There is a great deal to be said for discussing your ideas openly with your family. With no need for secrecy, members of the family can be involved if you want them to be. Your own resolve may be tested in the process, for you must be strong enough in your own conviction to override the objections that others may have. Avoidance of unnecessary suffering is usually the main reason to consider an earlier death, and your family must eventually accept that motive, if they are to know about your plans at all. You can ask your family to share in your suffering and understand your desire for release, requesting that they place your wishes ahead of their own. You must help them understand that the choice is not between life and death but between optional death sooner and compulsory death later. In making it clear that your desire to die sooner is for release from suffering and should not be viewed as rejection of a supportive family, you can pre-empt or at least minimize psychological harm to your loved ones.

Impending death is a strong stimulus for expressions of forgiveness, closeness, and love. It presents an opportunity to review your individual lives, your lives together, and what you have meant to each other. Such discussions help family members to deal with grief so that only sadness remains at the end: life goes on without the loved one who has died, but with a minimum of regret and guilt. This requires talking with each family member, in an open sharing of concerns and feelings, ideally one-on-one and at length. The value of this opportunity to communicate cannot be overestimated. Reassurance of love and understanding, forgiveness of actual or perceived slights, correction of misunderstandings, and fence mending can all take place in the days or weeks before death. Affection, bonding, and healing are part of the process. The hospice system emphasizes the value to the family of these last few days in the hospice environment, where family members are brought together for a meaningful farewell. In fact, any peaceful and reasonably private environment will do. The essential ingredients are not the environment but the acceptance of death and the desire to communicate. Assisted death in the familiar surroundings of one's own home is certainly as congenial as the hospice environment—more congenial, many would say. Obtaining assistance in dying decreases the uncertainty about when death will occur and puts real pressure on all who are immediately concerned to deal with the issue now rather than deferring it to some unknown and unwelcome future date.

Because of the difficulty that these discussions may present, the sooner your family hears your thoughts about assisted dying the better, ideally when you are alert and comfortable. They may not like the idea at all and you may have to talk them into accepting it. You can expect sorrows that must be soothed and differences of opinion that must be overcome, taking personal responsibility for your decision. In turn, they may talk you out of it. If they love you, it is understandable that they would like to have you around a little longer. But just as you must accept your own death, if you are going to deliberately shorten your life, your family must accept it, too. If you are terminally ill, the loss and hardship that will result from death cannot be avoided for long. A cancer patient told me of a note that she wrote to her family: "I know that I promised that I would do everything that I could in my power to get rid of the illness. I would go through all the treatments and all the chemo and all the radiation and all the operations and everything else. Now it's coming to the time where I'm asking you to release me from that promise and to let me go. If you really and truly love me, please say that you will set me free."

Some families are too estranged to participate in end-of-life decisions. The families of some AIDS patients are badly fractured, and divorces can alter loyalties. A person who wishes to exclude his family from any discussion of an earlier death should make this clear to his physician. Until laws are passed that clearly define patient autonomy in such situations, the physician who assists in death will be at risk of being sued by any member of the family who was left out of the discussion. As the laws change and assisted dying becomes legal, the agreement will become a much more personal one between patient and physician. Although it is still desirable to include some family, consent should never be required, nor should any member of the family have veto power over the wishes of the competent patient.

In my own hospital a sixty-year-old woman was brought to the emergency room with severe weakness and some respiratory difficulty from advanced leukemia. She asked the doctors not to intubate her, even though she was having trouble breathing. Her own physician was contacted and said that she was not expected to live long and could definitely be made DNR. Her family disagreed, however, and demanded that she be intubated. She was too depressed to know what she truly wanted, they insisted, and she shouldn't be listened to. Her daughter said, "Let me into the room and I'll talk her out of it." Because of the disagreement and her critical status, the patient was intubated, but she died twenty-four hours later. She had never discussed her wishes with her family, and they were not prepared to respect them in the emergency that developed.

Families can be seriously split if they are required to participate in end-of-life decisions. While most are brought closer together by helping their loved ones through a period of suffering, others find that the strain can be too great and has just the opposite effect. Terminal illness can bring out the worst as well as the best in people— including the extreme case, the family that deliberately encourages a person to consider an earlier death.

In some cultures the dying are insulated from the concept of death, much as they were in the United States fifty or sixty years ago.

Even when the person is completely competent, DNR orders, advance directives, and powers of attorney are not discussed with the patient. Those are "family decisions" that are traditionally made for, rather than by, the patient.[9] In our multicultural society, we should understand these differences and respect the rules of the family's culture rather than imposing our own.

The support of family and friends, though, can help some people face death with grace and even humor. A patient of mine described her husband's death in Jerusalem: "Outside of our apartment there was a beautiful flowering tree that we could see through the window. Shortly before he died my husband pointed it out to friends from his bed, 'Look at that lovely tree. In Israel you even get a preview.'"

Current laws forbidding physicians from assisting in dying create pressure for families to take on this responsibility themselves. In some gay communities, assisting partners or friends to die is fairly common. This practice may decline as physicians are allowed to take on more responsibility. Even while physician-assisted dying is illegal, the risks for the physician are probably much less than they are for any family member. Families can feel trapped by unthinkingly agreeing to help, only to find that the real challenge is much more than they expected. This is an excellent reason why the family needs to be supportive but must leave the actual help to the physician. Ideally, whether legal or not, assisted death should not take place alone. Family, physician, or friends should be present, individually or in some combination. But there is a significant difference between just being there and actually helping with the death, and it should be understood that direct help by family members will continue to be a crime, even after physician-assisted dying is legalized.

The controversy that surrounds assisted dying has encouraged many people to examine their own wishes more closely. We are in transit from a society that did not want to think about death at all to one that is increasingly concerned about how life may end. Far from being a step toward moral oblivion, assisted dying may in fact be a step uphill to a better society, which places greater value on life. It is doubtful that we are now at the absolute crest of our moral development in this area, so that the only way is down. If there is risk in going higher, we can certainly avail ourselves of the means to safeguard our journey. We have no need to be frozen with terror, unable to go up or down, for fear of causing an avalanche that will wipe out all that is good in humankind. The passage of compassionate laws will not bring about the end of our civilization any more than will the acts of compassionate physicians.

Notes

INTRODUCTION

Epigraph: Dissenting in *Cruzan v. Director, Missouri Department of Health*, 497 U.S. 261, 310–11 (1990).

1. *Compassion in Dying v. State of Washington*, 79 F.3d 790, 824 (9th Cir. 1996); *Compassion in Dying* 79 F.3d at 802.
2. Quotations from "U.S. Not Ready for Doctor-Executioner," *American Medical News*, November 25, 1991, p. 17.
3. A. Schopenhauer, "On Suicide, in Studies in Pessimism," in *Complete Essays of Schopenhauer*, trans. T. Bailey Saunders (New York: Wiley, 1942), 25.
4. D. W. Brock discussed this point in Medical Grand Rounds at Yale University on January 9, 1997.

CHAPTER 1. THE NEEDS OF THE PATIENT

1. D. J. Weatherall, editorial, *British Medical Journal* 309 (1994):1671–72.
2. L. R. Slome et al., "Physician Assisted Suicide and Patients with Human Immunodeficiency Virus Disease," *New Eng. J. Med.* 336 (1997):417–21.
3. N. L. Mace and P. V. Rabins, *The 36-Hour Day: A Family Guide to Caring for Persons with Alzheimer's Disease, Related Demented Illnesses, and Memory Loss in Later Life* (Baltimore: Johns Hopkins University Press, 1991).

4. G. M. McKhann, professor of neurology, director of the Mind Brain Institute, Johns Hopkins University, personal communication.

5. A. B. Lerner, "I've Lost a Kingdom: A Victim's Remarks on Alzheimer's Disease," *Connecticut Medicine* 58 (1991):281–82.

6. S. G. Post, "Alzheimer's Disease and the 'Then' Self," *Kennedy Institute of Ethics Journal* 5 (1995):307–21.

7. R. Dworkin, *Life's Dominion: An Argument About Abortion, Euthanasia, and Individual Freedom* (New York: Alfred A. Knopf, 1993), 221.

8. D. Callahan, "Terminating Life: Sustaining Treatment of the Demented," *Hastings Center Report* 25 (1995):29.

9. R. Dresser, "Dworkin on Dementia: Elegant Theory, Questionable Policy," *Hastings Center Report* 25 (1995):35.

10. Dr. Audrey Heimler is a University of Connecticut genetic counselor for families with Huntington's disease. She was very helpful in providing information about this illness. Similarly, John Halleran, director of the Sterling Manor Nursing Home, was very helpful in showing me his facility and explaining the management and financial aspects of caring for patients with Alzheimer's and Huntington's diseases.

11. Quotation from D. Clendinen, "When Death Is a Blessing and Life Is Not," *New York Times,* February 5, 1996.

12. L. Stevens, "For an Ill Widow, 83, Suicide Is Welcome," *New York Times,* August 2, 1989.

13. M. P. Battin, "Is There a Duty to Die? Age Rationing and the Just Distribution of Health Care," chap. 3 in *The Least Worst Death: Essays in Bioethics on the End of Life* (New York: Oxford University Press, 1994).

14. D. Callahan and M. White, "The Legalization of Physician-Assisted Suicide: Creating a Regulatory Potemkin Village," *U. of Richmond Law Rev.* 30 (1996):11–12.

15. P. J. van der Maas et al., *Euthanasia and Other Medical Decisions Concerning the End of Life* (London: Elsevier Amsterdam, 1992), 45.

16. Dworkin, *Life's Dominion,* 238.

17. J. Fletcher, *Humanhood: Essays in Biomedical Ethics* (Buffalo, N.Y.: Prometheus, 1979).

18. E. Cassell, "The Function of Medicine," *Hastings Center Report* 27 (1977), 16–19.

19. D. Callahan, "When Self-Determination Runs Amok," in *Life Choices: A Hastings Center Introduction to Bioethics,* ed. J. H. Howell and W. F. Sale (Washington, D.C.: Georgetown University Press, 1995), 249.

20. H. Kuhse, *The Sanctity-of-Life Doctrine in Medicine: A Critique* (Oxford: Clarendon, 1987).

21. Justice Cardozo, *Schloendorff v. New York Hospital* 211 N.Y. 125, 129, 105 N.E. 92, 93 (1914).

22. A case in medical futility went to court in Minnesota in 1995. Helga Wanglie was eighty-five years old when she was admitted to a hospital in Minneapolis after sustaining a hip fracture. In the hospital she had many medical problems, including a cardiopulmonary arrest, which left her in a persistent vegetative state on a respirator. Her condition was deemed hopeless, and further treatment regarded as futile by all of those caring for her. Her husband, however, requested that all treatment be continued despite the bleak outlook. The hospital petitioned the court to be allowed to discontinue Mrs. Wanglie's support. The court sided with Mr. Wanglie, though, and appointed him as his wife's conservator. See J. F. Daar, "Medical Futility and Implications for Physician Autonomy," *Am. J. Law and Med.* 21 (1995):221–40.

23. L. Kass, "Neither for Love nor Money: Why Doctors Must Not Kill," *Public Interest* 94 (1989):25–46.

24. D. J. Bakker, "Active Euthanasia: Is Mercy Killing the Killing of Mercy?" in *Euthanasia: The Good of the Patient, the Good of Society,* ed. R. I. Misbin (Frederick, Md.: University Publishing Group, 1992), 88.

25. D. Callahan, *The Troubled Dream of Life: Living with Mortality* (New York: Simon and Schuster, 1993), 106.

26. T. R. Fried et al., "Limits of Patient Autonomy: Physicians' Attitudes and Practices Regarding Life-Sustaining Treatments and Euthanasia," *Archives of Internal Medicine* 153 (1993): 722–28.

27. I am indebted to the following people for providing information on medical and welfare finances as they affect patients and families: Cheryl Vann, coordinator for Title 19 patients at Yale–New Haven Hospital (YNHH); Bonnie Indeck, social services department, YNHH; Virginia Roddy, attorney in risk management office of YNHH; Susan Nobleman, attorney for elderly in Hamden, Connecticut; B. Kaliszewski, State of Connecticut, Department of Social Services; and Leslie Walker Broceland, Center for Mental Health and Aging in Connecticut.

28. Theodore R. Marmor, professor of public management, Yale School of Management, personal communication, 1997.

29. *Compassion in Dying v. State of Washington,* 79 F.3d 790, 826 (9th Cir. 1996).

CHAPTER 2. RATIONAL SUICIDE

Epigraph: "Apologia for Suicide," in *Euthanasia and the Right to Die: The Case for Voluntary Euthanasia,* ed. A. B. Downing (London: Peter Owen, 1969),

154. Barrington is an attorney who helped draft the Voluntary Euthanasia bill in England.

1. G. C. Graber, "Mastering the Concept of Suicide," in *Suicide, Right or Wrong?* ed. J. Donnelly (Buffalo, N.Y.: Prometheus, 1990).

2. R. B. Brandt, "The Morality and Rationality of Suicide," in Donnelly, *Suicide, Right or Wrong?* 185.

3. M. Stauch, "Rationality and the Refusal of Medical Treatment: A Critique of the Recent Approach of the English Courts," *J. Med. Ethics* 21 (1995): 162–65.

4. E. S. Shneidman, "Some Essentials of Suicide and Some Implications for Responses," in *Suicide,* ed. A. Roy (Baltimore: Williams and Wilkins, 1986), 1–16.

5. J. P. Tupin, "Psychiatric Issues of Euthanasia," in *Beneficent Euthanasia,* ed. M. Kohl (Buffalo, N.Y.: Prometheus, 1975).

6. A. Kerkhof, associate professor of social and behavioral science, Department of Clinical Health and Personality Psychology, Leiden University, the Netherlands, interview, June 1995.

7. Y. Kamisar, "Euthanasia Legislation: Some Non-Religious Objections," in Downing, *Euthanasia and the Right to Die,* 92.

8. S. Freud, "Thoughts for the Times on War and Death," in *The Standard Edition of the Complete Psychological Works of Sigmund Freud* 14, trans. and ed. J. Strachey (London: Hogarth, 1953), 289.

9. L. J. Markson et al., "Physician Assessment of Patient Competence," *J. Am. Geriatric Soc.* 42 (1994):1074.

10. Ibid.

11. Y. Conwell, and E. D. Caine, "Rational Suicide and the Right to Die: Reality and Myth," *New Eng. J. Med.* 325 (1991):1100–1103.

12. G. M. Burnell, "Psychiatric Assessment of the Suicidal Terminally Ill," *Hawaii Med. J.* 54 (1995):510–13. James Ciarcia is associate clinical professor of psychiatry at Yale University. His background includes fellowships at Memorial Sloan–Kettering Cancer Center in New York and the Sidney Farber Cancer Center in Boston. He is a consultant for Connecticut Hospice.

13. G. E. Valliant and S. J. Blumenthal, "Suicide over the Life Cycle: Risk Factors and Life-Span Development," in *Suicide over the Life Cycle: Risk Factors, Assessment, and Treatment of Suicidal Patients,* ed. S. J. Blumenthal and D. J. Kupfer (Washington, D.C.: American Psychiatric Press, 1990), 1–16.

14. Conwell and Caine, "Rational Suicide and the Right to Die."

15. Kerkhof interview.

16. H. Hendin, *Suicide in America* (New York: W. W. Norton, 1982), 215.

17. J. Fletcher, "Attitudes Towards Suicide," in Donnelly, *Suicide, Right or Wrong?*

18. L. Edelstein, in *Ancient Medicine: Selected Papers of Ludwig Edelstein,* ed. O. Temkin and C. L. Temkin (Baltimore: Johns Hopkins University Press, 1987).

19. Quoted in M. D. Sullivan and S. J. Youngner, "Depression, Competence, and the Right to Refuse Life-Saving Medical Treatment," *Am. J. Psych.* 151 (1994):971.

20. For a full discussion see R. Gillon, "Suicide and Voluntary Euthanasia: Historical Perspectives," in Downing, *Euthanasia and the Right to Die.*

21. C. S. Campbell, "Sovereignty, Stewardship and the Self: Religious Perspectives on Euthanasia," in *Euthanasia: The Good of the Patient, The Good of Society,* ed. R. I. Misbin (Frederick, Md.: University Publishing Group, 1992).

22. Ibid. These summaries were updated from those published by Campbell.

23. General Assembly of the Unitarian Universalist Association, "The Right to Die with Dignity: 1988," *Resolutions and Resources,* ed. K. Devine and M. Rosa (Boston: 1990), 74.

24. The Presbyterian General Assembly has discussed but has not taken a stand on assisted dying. A retired minister, Gaspar Langella of Jasper, Georgia, wrote an article for a study group convened by the Park Ridge Center in 1992–93, "The Voluntary Active Euthanasia and Physician Assisted Suicide Question: Public Policy Consideration from a Reformed-Presbyterian Point of View." Langella states that judgment should favor a person's choice and that there is continuing need for public discussion.

25. This summary of Jewish teaching is based on a discussion with Rabbi Michael Whitman of Young Israel Temple of New Haven.

26. For a comprehensive review of the Catholic position against suicide and euthanasia, some of which is summarized here, see R. L. Barry, *Breaking the Thread of Life* (New Brunswick N.J.: Transaction, 1994). This book draws heavily on Catholic teachings and doctrine and frequently considers all suicide together, rather that separating out those associated with underlying terminal illness and suffering.

27. St. Augustine, *The City of God.*

28. St. Thomas Aquinas, *Summa Theologica.*

29. American Lutheran Church, *Health, Life, and Death: A Christian Perspective* (Minneapolis, Minn.: Office of Church and Society, 1977).

30. J. Sullivan, *Catholic Teaching on the Morality of Euthanasia* (Washington, D.C.: Catholic University of America, 1949).

31. Barry, *Breaking the Thread of Life,* 149–50.

32. H. Kuhse, *The Sanctity-of-Life Doctrine in Medicine: A Critique* (Oxford: Clarendon, 1987).

33. M. P. Battin, *Ethical Issues in Suicide* (Englewood Cliffs, N.J.: Prentice Hall, 1995), 208.

34. W. R. Matthews, "Voluntary Euthanasia: The Ethical Aspect," in Downing, *Euthanasia and the Right to Die,* 25–29.

35. D. Maguire, "A Catholic View on Mercy Killing," in Kohl, *Beneficent Euthanasia.*

36. Cited by M. P. Battin, in *The Least Worst Death: Essays in Bioethics on the End of Life* (New York: Oxford University Press, 1994), 244.

37. C. S. Campbell, "Sovereignty, Stewardship, and the Self: Religious Perspectives on Euthanasia," in Misbin, *Euthanasia.*

38. G. Williams, *The Sanctity of Life and the Criminal Law* (New York: Alfred A. Knopf, 1972), 258–59.

39. Sir William Blackstone, *Commentaries on the Laws of England: 1765–69.*

40. Cited by M. Angell, "Prisoners of Technology: The Case of Nancy Cruzan," *New Eng. J. Med.* 322 (1990):1226.

41. Anthony Lewis reported in "Perchance to Dream," an op-ed piece in the *New York Times,* January 10, 1970, that on September 21, 1939, Freud told his physician, Dr. Max Schur: "My Dear Schur, you certainly remember our first talk. You promised then not to forsake me when my time comes. Now it's nothing but torture and makes no sense anymore."

42. *Vital Statistics for the United States* (1996).

43. N. A. Pace, "We Should Treat Depression, Not Assist Suicide," *New York Times,* February 4, 1993.

44. Sullivan and Youngner, "Depression, Competence, and the Right to Refuse Life-Saving Medical Treatment," 971.

45. Ciarcia, interview.

46. E. Emanuel et al., "Euthanasia and Physician-Assisted Suicide: Attitudes and Experiences of Oncology Patients, Oncologists, and the Public," *Lancet* 347 (1996):1805–10.

47. J. H. Brown, P. Henteleff, S. Barakat, and C. J. Rowe, "Is It Normal for Terminally Ill Patients to Desire Death?" *Am. J. Psych.* 143 (1986):208.

48. A. Solomon, "A Death of One's Own," *New Yorker,* May 22, 1995, 54–69.

CHAPTER 3. THE SEARCH FOR HELP

1. A directive can also be given that every effort be made to extend the patient's life as long as possible. This brings up another aspect of medical futility. In one noteworthy case, a court granted a man the right to keep his comatose

wife on an artificial support system against the advice of the hospital and the physicians involved. See Chapter 1, note 22.

2. D. Orentlicher, "The Illusion of Patient Choice in End-of-Life Decisions," *J. Am. Med. Assoc.* 267 (1992):2101–4. Orentlicher represents the Office of the General Counsel, American Medical Association.

3. Support Principle Investigators, "A Controlled Trial to Improve Care for Seriously Ill, Hospitalized Patients: The Study to Understand Prognosis and Preferences for Outcomes and Risks of Treatments (SUPPORT)," *J. Am. Med. Assoc.* 274 (1995):1591–98.

4. I am indebted to the following people for discussing the hospice program with me: Rosemary Hertzler, R.N., director of Connecticut Hospice; Fred Flatow, M.D., staff physician at Connecticut Hospice; Robert Donaldson, M.D., visiting physician at Connecticut Hospice; Cathy Sumpio, R.N., staff nurse at Connecticut Hospice; and Ginger Davidson, R.N., Mary Carney, R.N., and Mary Thieren, R.N., home hospice nurses in Connecticut.

5. T. M. Stephany, "Physician Assisted Euthanasia Is Necessary," in *Euthanasia: Opposing Viewpoints,* ed. Carol Wekesser (San Diego: Greenhaven, 1995), 111. Theresa Stephany is a hospice nurse.

6. R. J. Miller, "Hospice Care as an Alternative to Euthanasia," *Law, Med., and Health Care* 20 (1992):127–32.

7. I am indebted to the following people for discussing the Hemlock Society with me: Midge Levy, Hemlock Society of Washington State; Faye Girsh, executive director of Hemlock Society, USA; and John Pridonoff, former executive director of Hemlock Society, USA.

8. D. Humphrey, *Final Exit: The Practicalities of Self-Deliverance and Assisted Suicide for the Dying* (Eugene, Ore.: Hemlock Society, 1991).

9. I am indebted to the following people for discussing the Compassion in Dying program with me: Rev. Ralph Mero, Seattle, founder of Compassion in Dying; Susan Dunshee and Thomas Preston, M.D., members of Compassion in Dying; and Kathryn Tucker of the law firm of Perkins Coie, Seattle, attorney for Compassion in Dying, who represented cases from New York and Washington State to the Second and Ninth Circuit Courts of Appeal and to the U.S. Supreme Court.

10. Compassion in Dying's services and procedures are well described in L. Belkin, "There's No Simple Suicide," *New York Times Magazine,* November 14, 1993, p. 48.

11. T. E. Quill, "Death and Dignity: A Case of Individualized Decision Making," *New Eng. J. Med.* 324 (1991):691–94.

12. T. E. Quill, *Death and Dignity: Making Choices and Taking Charge* (New

York: W. W. Norton, 1993); T. E. Quill, *A Midwife Through the Dying Process* (Baltimore: Johns Hopkins University Press, 1996).

13. R. J. Blendon et al., "Should Physicians Aid Their Patients in Dying? The Public Perspective," *J. Am. Med. Assoc.* 267 (1992):2658–62.

14. J. A. Jacobson et al., "Decedents' Reported Preferences for Physician Assisted Death: A Survey of Informants Listed on Death Certificates in Utah," *J. Med. Ethics* 6 (1995):149–57.

15. D. P. Caddell and R. R. Newton, "Euthanasia: American Attitudes Toward the Physician's Role," *Soc. Sci. Med.* 40 (1995):1671–81.

16. E. Emanuel, "The History of Euthanasia Debates in the United States and Britain," *Ann. of Int. Med.* 121 (1994):793–802. See also E. J. Emanuel et al., "Euthanasia and Physician-Assisted Suicide: Attitudes and Experiences of Oncology Patients, Oncologists, and the Public," *Lancet* 347(1996): 1805–10.

17. Quill, "Death and Dignity"; L. Kass, "Neither for Love nor Money: Why Doctors Must Not Kill," *Public Interest* 94 (1989):25–46.

18. See A. C. Mermann, D. B. Gunn, and G. E. Dickinson, "Learning to Care for the Dying: A Survey of Medical Schools and a Model Course," *Acad. Med.* 66 (1991):35–38.

19. P. V. Caralis, and J. S. Hammond, "Attitudes of Medical Students, Housestaff, and Faculty Physicians Toward Euthanasia and Termination of Life Sustaining Treatment," *Critical Care Med.* 20 (1992):683–90.

20. The Massachusetts Medical Society, in collaboration with the *Boston Globe,* contacted 837 physicians who care for dying patients. Twenty-one percent had received requests and 19 percent had helped patients die. Forty-three percent thought that some form of physician-assisted dying should be legalized, and 53 percent said that they would do it if it were legal. Dick Lehr, "Death and the Doctor's Hand," *Boston Globe,* April 25–27, 1993. In a similar study Ezekial Emanuel of the Dana Farber Center contacted 350 oncologists nationwide. More than half had received requests for physician-assisted suicide and 37 percent for euthanasia. Thirteen percent had assisted suicide and 2 percent with euthanasia. Emanuel et al., "Euthanasia and Physician-Assisted Suicide." A similar study in Washington State, where a recently defeated referendum proposal focused attention on the subject, showed that 53 percent of 938 physicians contacted were in favor of laws that would permit assisted suicide and that 40 percent would participate if it were legal. The figures for euthanasia were 53 percent and 33 percent, respectively. J. S. Cohen et al., "Attitudes Toward Assisted Suicide and Euthanasia Among Physicians in Washington State," *New Eng. J. Med.* 331

(1994):89–94. In Oregon, also the site of considerable recent public debate on assisted dying, 60 percent of physicians thought that assisted suicide should be legal and 46 percent would be willing to participate if it was. M. A. Lee et al., "Legalizing Assisted Suicide: Views of Physicians in Oregon," *New Eng. J. Med.* 334 (1996):310–15. Figures for New Jersey were similar, with 50 percent of physicians in favor of assisted suicide and 36 percent willing to participate. M. Reisner and A. N. Damato, "Attitudes of Physicians Regarding Physician Assisted Suicide," *New Jer. Med.* 92, no. 10 (1995):663–66. Physicians in Michigan have had heavy exposure to this issue through legal attempts to restrict Dr. Kevorkian. A survey was carried out of all of the oncologists in that state. Responses were received from 154 of 250 in practice. Thirty-eight percent had received requests for assisted suicide, and 18 percent had provided assistance. Forty-three percent had received requests for euthanasia and 4 percent had honored them. D. J. Doukas et al., "Attitudes and Behaviors on Physician-Assisted Death: A Study of Michigan Oncologists," *J. Clin. Oncol.* 13 (1995):1055–61. In a broader poll, 54 percent of Michigan physicians thought that physician-assisted suicide should be legal, and 35 percent thought they would participate if it were. J. G. Bachman et al., "Attitudes of Michigan Physicians and the Public Toward Legalizing Physician Assisted Suicide and Voluntary Euthanasia," *New Eng. J. Med.* 334 (1996):303–9. The California referendum question in 1988, entitled "The Humane and Dignified Death Act," was initially opposed by the California Medical Association. The San Francisco Medical Society, however, found that 70 percent of responding members thought that "patients should have the option of requesting active euthanasia when faced with incurable, terminal illness," and 45 percent said they would participate if it were legal. S. Helig, "The SFMS Euthanasia Survey: Results and Analysis," *San Francisco Medicine,* May 1988, pp. 24–26. A survey of National Health Service physicians in one area of England showed that 163 out of 273 had been asked at some time to hasten death and that 32 percent had complied, representing 12 percent of the respondents. Moreover, 46 percent would consider helping to bring about death if it were legal. B. J. Ward and P. A. Tate, "Attitudes Among NHS Doctors to Requests for Euthanasia," *Brit. Med. J.* 308 (1994):1332–34.

21. S. H. Wanzer et al., "The Physician's Responsibility Towards Hopelessly Ill Patients: A Second Look," *New Eng. J. Med.* 320 (1989):844–49. The conference that led to this article was convened by the Society for the Right to Die and was held at Harvard Medical School in October 1987.

22. G. Kolata, "1 in 5 Nurses Tell Survey They Helped Patients Die," *New York*

Times, May 23, 1996; A. Young et al., "Oncology Nurses' Attitudes Regarding Voluntary, Physician Assisted Dying for Competent, Terminally Ill Patients," *Oncology Nursing Forum* 20 (1993):445–51.

23. L. J. Schneiderman and R. G. Spragg, "Ethical Decisions in Discontinuing Mechanical Ventilation," *New Eng. J. Med.* 318 (1988):984–88.

24. The Roman Catholic Church is still divided on the issue of ordinary versus extraordinary treatment or supportive measures. See W. E. May, "Comment on Nutrition and Hydration: Moral Considerations, a Statement of the Catholic Bishops of Pennsylvania," *Linacre Quarterly,* February 1992, pp. 34–36; P. Steinfels, "Bishops Warn Against Withdrawing Life Supports," *New York Times,* April 3, 1992. A good discussion is also presented by G. M. Craig, "On Withholding Nutrition and Hydration in the Terminally Ill: Has Palliative Medicine Gone Too Far?" *J. Med. Ethics* 20 (1994):138–43.

25. J. L. Bernat et al., "Patient Refusal of Hydration and Nutrition: An Alternative to Physician-Assisted Suicide or Voluntary Active Euthanasia," *Archives Internal Medicine* 153 (1993):2723–28.

26. R. M. McCann, W. J. Hall, et al., "Comfort Care of Terminally Ill Patients: The Appropriate Use of Nutrition and Hydration," *J. Am. Med. Assoc.* 272 (1994):1263–66.

27. In Holland the most commonly used drugs are Nembutol and Seconal, taken at a dose of nine grams (ninety capsules) in three to four ounces of fluid.

28. Presumably mindful of the fact that the penalty for murder is much greater than that for assisting suicide, Kevorkian has always used devices that were activated by the patients.

29. In Holland the most commonly used drugs are Pentothal, at a dose of twenty milligrams per kilogram of body weight, followed by twenty milligrams of Pavalon.

30. D. T. Watts and T. Howell, "Assisted Suicide Is Not Euthanasia," *J. Am. Geriatric Soc.* 40 (1992):1043.

31. H. Brody, "Assisted Death: A Compassionate Response to Medical Failure," *New Eng. J. Med.* 327 (1992):1384–88.

32. Fye, "Permissive Euthanasia," *Boston Med. and Surg. J.* (now *New Eng. J. Med.*) (1884):501-2. Cited in "When Death Is Sought: Assisted Suicide and Euthanasia in the Medical Context," New York State Task Force on Life and the Law, 1994, 112, ref. 123.

33. D. Orentlicher, "The Legalization of Physician-Assisted Suicide," *New Eng. J. Med.* 335 (1996):663–67.

34. C. H. Baron, "The Functional Distinction Between Active and Passive Euthanasia and the Danger It Poses to the Civil Liberties of Patients," speech

delivered at the Biennial Conference of the American Civil Liberties Union, June 26–30, 1991, at the University of Vermont. Charles Baron is professor of law, Boston College Law School.

35. J. Rachels, "Active and Passive Euthanasia," *New Eng. J. Med.* 294 (1975): 78–80. See also J. Rachels, *End of Life: Euthanasia and Morality* (New York: Oxford University Press, 1986).

36. *Quill v. Vocco,* 80 F. 3d, 716 (2d Cir. 1996).

37. Religious and ethical aspects of the rules of double effect are discussed extensively in *Principles of Biomedical Ethics,* 4th ed., ed. T. L. Beauchamp and J. F. Childress (New York: Oxford University Press, 1994), 206–11; and R. F. Weir, *Abating Treatment with Critically Ill Patients* (New York: Oxford University Press, 1989).

38. N. L. Cantor and G. C. Thomas, "Pain Relief, Acceleration of Death, and Criminal Law," *Kennedy Inst. of Ethics J.* 6 (1996):107–27.

39. T. A. Preston, "Killing Pain, Ending Life," *New York Times,* November 1, 1994. Preston, a cardiologist and professor of medicine at the University of Washington, is also one of the founders of Compassion in Dying.

40. T. E. Quill, R. Dresser, and D. W. Brock, "The Rule of Double Effect: A Critique of Its Role in End-of-Life Decision Making," *New Eng. J. Med.* 337 (1997):1768–71.

41. D. Orentlicher, "The Supreme Court Decision and Physician Assisted Suicide: Rejecting Assisted Suicide but Embracing Euthanasia," *New Eng. J. Med.* 337 (1997):1236–39.

CHAPTER 4. DYING ALONE OR DYING WITH HELP

1. A. C. Cain, *Survivors of Suicide* (Springfield, Ill.: Charles C. Thomas, 1972).

2. J. Legemaate, "Legal Aspects of Euthanasia and Assisted Suicide in the Netherlands, 1973–1994," in *Euthanasia in the Netherlands,* 3d ed. (Royal Dutch Medical Association, 1994), 38.

3. T. H. C. Bueller, "The Historical and Religious Framework for Euthanasia in the Netherlands," in *Euthanasia: The Good of the Patient, The Good of Society,* ed. R. I. Misbin (Frederick, Md.: University Publishing Group, 1992).

4. T. M. G. van Berkestijan, "The Royal Dutch Medical Association and the Practice of Euthanasia and Assisted Suicide," in *Euthanasia in the Netherlands,* 27–36. Berkestijan was the secretary general of the Royal Dutch Medical Association.

5. M. P. Battin, "A Dozen Caveats Concerning the Discussion of Euthanasia in the Netherlands," in *The Least Worst Death,* ed. M. P. Battin (New York: Oxford University Press, 1994).

6. W. S. van Oijen, interview, June 1995. Dr. Wilfred S. van Oijen is a family practitioner in Amsterdam who has assisted in several deaths, including the one recorded for the television documentary *Death on Request.*

7. *Euthanasia in the Netherlands,* 39–40. These guidelines are discussed in detail in Chapter 7.

8. An astonishing extension of the rules of eligibility permitted euthanasia for a psychiatric patient suffering from chronic severe depression requiring numerous hospitalizations. The patient made several requests for assisted dying and eventually received it.

9. M. P. Battin, "Should We Copy the Dutch? The Netherlands' Practice of Voluntary Euthanasia as a Model for the United States," in Misbin, *Euthanasia;* H. Kuhse, "Voluntary Euthanasia in the Netherlands," *Med. J. of Australia* 147 (1987):394–96; S. H. Wanzer et al., "The Physician's Responsibility Toward Hopelessly Ill Patients: A Second Look," *New Eng. J. Med.* 320 (1989):844; T. E. Quill, *Death and Dignity: Making Choices and Taking Charge* (New York: W. W. Norton, 1993), 146–51. The widely quoted Wanzer article was cowritten by ten medical and legal scholars, eight of whom support some form of assisted dying under appropriate conditions.

10. C. F. Gomez, *Regulating Death: Euthanasia and the Case of the Netherlands* (New York: Free Press, 1991); A. M. Capron, "Euthanasia in the Netherlands: American Observations," *Hastings Center Report* 22 (1992):32; R. Fenigsen, "A Case against Dutch Euthanasia," *Hastings Center Report* 19 (1989):S26.

11. P. J. van der Maas, J. J. M. van Delden, L. Pijnenborg, et al., "Euthanasia and Other Medical Decisions Concerning the End of Life," *Lancet* 338 (1991):669–74; G. van der Wal et al., "Euthanasia and Assisted Suicide: How Often Is It Practiced by Family Doctors in the Netherlands?" *Family Practice* 9 (1992):130–34. The full text of the van der Maas article was published in *Health Policy Monograph* 2 (Amsterdam: Elsevier, 1992). Paul van der Maas is professor in the department of public health of the Medical Facility of Erasmus University, Rotterdam. Van der Wal is inspector of public health for the province of North Holland, Haarlem. *Euthanasia* in Dutch terminology is limited to what we in the United States consider active voluntary euthanasia.

12. L. Pijnenborg, P. J. van der Maas, et al., "Life-Terminating Acts Without Explicit Request of Patient," *Lancet* 341 (1993):1196–99.

13. This is a marked improvement over the rates of reporting of 3 percent in 1986 and 17 percent in 1990. G. van der Wal and R. J. M. Dillmann, "Euthanasia in the Netherlands," *Brit. Med. J.* 308 (May 21, 1994):1346.

14. G. van der Wal, interview, June 1995.

15. H. J. J. Leenen, "Euthanasia in the Netherlands," in *Medicine, Medical Ethics, and the Value of Life,* ed. P. Byrne (London: John Wiley and Sons, 1990), 1–14.

CHAPTER 5. PHYSICIANS' CONCERNS

Epigraph: "The Principle of Euthanasia," in *Euthanasia and the Right to Die: The Case for Voluntary Euthanasia,* ed. A. B. Downing (London: Peter Owen, 1969), 36.

1. J. Rachels, *The End of Life: Euthanasia and Morality* (New York: Oxford University Press, 1986), 163.

2. H. Feifel, "Death," in *Taboo Topics,* ed. N. L. Farberow (New York: Atherton, 1963).

3. A medical oncologist explained that patient withdrawal and depression may be cultural, based in particular on her experiences with Italian and Jewish patients. She cited one patient who seemed to lose the will to live: "We offered her chemotherapy, so she had to know her diagnosis. She is now really sitting there waiting to die. I don't see how we as physicians, or even the entire health care team, can change it. It is a cultural thing, and we never should have told her she had cancer in the first place."

4. G. J. Annas, "Informed Consent, Cancer, and Truth in Prognosis," *New Eng. J. Med.* 330 (1994):223–25.

5. M. Angell, "Respecting the Autonomy of Competent Patients," *New Eng. J. Med.* 310 (1984):1115–16.

6. Ibid.

7. The heavy burden that helping a person to die imposes on the physician is well described by two physicians who disconnected a ventilator at the request of a patient who knew he would die. M. J. Edwards and S. W. Tolle, "Disconnecting a Ventilator at the Request of a Patient Who Knows He Will Then Die: A Doctor's Anguish," *Ann. of Int. Med.* 117 (1992):254–56. The anguish is also expressed by a renal specialist who declined to shorten by a few days the life of a patient who had already discontinued dialysis. C. M. Kjellstrand, "The Impossible Choice," *J. Am. Med. Assoc.* 257 (1987):233.

8. T. L. Beauchamp and J. F. Childress, *Principles of Biomedical Ethics,* 4th ed. (New York: Oxford University Press, 1994), 470–74.

9. L. Kass, "Neither for Love nor Money: Why Doctors Must Not Kill," *Public Interest* 94 (1989):25–46.

10. F. G. Miller and H. Brody, "Professional Integrity and Physician Assisted Death," *Hastings Center Report* 25 (1995):8–17.

11. S. H. Miles, "Physician Assisted Suicide and the Profession's Gyrocompass," *Hastings Center Report* 25 (1995):17–19.

12. P. Carrick, *Medical Ethics in Antiquity: Philosophical Perspectives on Abortion and Euthanasia* (Dordrecht: D. Reidel, 1985).

13. H. Wolinsky and T. Brune, "The Abortion Crisis," in *The Serpent on the Staff: The Unhealthy Politics of the AMA* (New York: G. P. Putnam's Sons, 1994).

14. T. A. Preston, "Professional Norms and Physician Attitudes Towards Euthanasia," *J. of Law, Med., and Ethics* 22 (1994):36–40. In spite of dissension within the ranks of the AMA or other national and state medical societies, the organizations speak with strong voices. Thomas Preston, a physician in Seattle who has been one of the major forces behind the Compassion in Dying movement, thinks that many physicians who are sympathetic to the goals of that organization stop short of publicly supporting physician-assisted dying because of fear of criticism by their colleagues and particularly by their medical society.

15. American Medical Association Council on Medical and Judicial Affairs, "Decisions Near the End of Life," *J. Am. Med. Assoc.* 267 (1992):2229–33.

16. C. K. Cassel and D. E. Meier, "Morals and Moralism in the Debate over Euthanasia and Assisted Suicide," *New Eng. J. Med.* 323 (1990):751.

17. D. Orentlicher, "Physician Participation in Assisted Suicide," *J. Am. Med. Assoc.* 262 (1989):1844–45. Subsequent writings by Orentlicher suggest that this was the official view of the AMA, which he did not personally share.

18. R. C. McMillan, "Responsibility *To* or *For* in the Physician-Patient Relationship?" *J. Med. Ethics* 21 (1995):112–15.

19. American Medical Association Council, "Decisions Near the End of Life."

20. Beauchamp and Childress, *Principles of Biomedical Ethics,* 5–6.

21. E. D. Pellegrino, "Compassion Needs Reason Too," *J. Am. Med. Assoc.* 270 (1993):874–75.

22. E. D. Pellegrino and D. Thomasma, *For the Patient's Good: The Restoration of Beneficence in Health Care* (New York: Oxford University Press, 1988), 29.

23. D. Callahan, *The Troubled Dream of Life: Living with Mortality* (New York: Simon and Schuster, 1993), 106.

24. H. Brody, *The Healer's Power* (New Haven: Yale University Press, 1992), 82.

25. Kass, "Neither for Love nor Money."

26. M. Angell, "Doctors and Assisted Suicide," *Annals RCPSC* 24 (1991): 94–95.

27. D. Meier, "Physician Assisted Dying: Theory and Reality," *J. Clin. Ethics* 3 (1992):35–37.

CHAPTER 6. PUBLIC CONCERNS

Epigraphs: Sullivan quoted in J. Rachels, *The End of Life: Euthanasia and Morality* (New York: Oxford University Press, 1986), 171; Woolman, *Journal* (New York: E. P. Dutton, 1910), cited by W. L. Sperry in the *Ethical Basis of Medical Practice* (London: Cassell, 1951). Willard Sperry, dean of Harvard Divinity School, gave a series of lectures on medical ethics at the Massachusetts General Hospital which were later published in his book. One of the lectures discussed physician-assisted dying.

1. Y. Kamisar, "Euthanasia Legislation: Some Non-Religious Objections," in *Euthanasia and the Right to Die,* ed. A. B. Downing (London: Peter Owen, 1969), 98–106.

2. P. J. van der Maas et al., "Euthanasia, Physician Assisted Suicide, and Other Medical Practices Involving the End of Life in the Netherlands, 1990–1995," *New Eng. J. Med.* 335 (1996):1699–1700. In Holland, where both assisted suicide and euthanasia are practiced, fewer than 0.5 percent of all deaths are from assisted suicide.

3. E. D. Pellegrino, "Compassion Needs Reason Too," *J. Am. Med. Assoc.* 270 (1993):874–76.

4. "Euthanasia enthusiasts" is from M. P. Battin, "Voluntary Euthanasia and the Risks of Abuse: Can We Learn Anything from the Netherlands?" *Law, Med., and Health Care* 20 (1992):136.

5. R. Doerflinger, "Assisted Suicide: Pro-Choice or Anti-Life," in *Life Choices: A Hastings Center Introduction to Bioethics,* ed. J. H. Howell and W. F. Sale (Washington, D.C.: Georgetown University Press, 1995), 247.

6. M. E. Gornick et al., "Effects of Race and Income on Mortality and Use of Services Among Medicare Beneficiaries," *New Eng. J. Med.* 335 (1996):791–99.

7. Y. Kamisar, "Against Assisted Suicide: Even a Very Limited Form," *U. Det. Mercy L. Rev.* 72 (1995):738.

8. See T. E. Quill, C. K. Cassel, and D. E. Meier, "Care of the Hopelessly Ill: Proposed Clinical Criteria for Physician Assisted Suicide," *New Eng. J. Med.* 327 (1992):1380–83; C. H. Baron et al., "A Model State Act to Authorize and Regulate Physician Assisted Suicide," *Harvard J. on Legislation* 33 (1996):1–34; F. G. Miller, T. E. Quill, et al., "Regulating Physician Assisted Death," *New Eng. J. Med.* 331 (1994):119–23; Battin, "Voluntary Euthanasia and the Risks of Abuse."

9. Quill et al., "Care of the Hopelessly Ill," 1381.

10. A Dutch physician, Pieter Admiraal, who was one of the first to practice assisted dying in that country, is an anesthesiologist.

11. Respectively, P. A. Singer and M. Siegler, "Euthanasia: A Critique," *New Eng. J. Med.* 322 (1990):1883; J. Lynn, Letter to Editor, *New Eng. J. Med.* 328 (1993):964.

12. D. Callahan and M. White, "The Legalization of Physician-Assisted Suicide: Creating a Regulatory Potemkin Village," *U. of Richmond Law Rev.* 30 (1996):3.

13. Pellegrino, "Compassion Needs Reason Too."

14. R. Doerflinger, "Assisted Suicide," 243.

15. D. Callahan, "When Self-Determination Runs Amok," *Hastings Center Report* 22 (1992):54. Kamisar ("Euthanasia Legislation") offers more of the same: "The reason why the 'parade of horrors' argument cannot be too lightly dismissed . . . is that the parade *has* taken place in our time, and the order of procession has been headed by the killing of 'incurables' and the 'useless.'"

16. Rachels, *End of Life,* 172–75.

17. M. P. Battin, "Fiction as Forecast: Euthanasia in Alzheimer's Disease," chap. 7 in *The Least Worst Death* (New York: Oxford University Press, 1994); and R. Dworkin, "Life Past Reason," chap. 8 in *Life's Dominion: An Argument About Abortion, Euthanasia, and Individual Freedom* (New York: Alfred A. Knopf, 1993).

18. J. A. Burgess, "The Great Slippery-Slope Argument," *J. Med. Ethics* 9 (1993):171.

19. Quotation from American Medical Association Council on Ethical and Judicial Affairs, *J. Am. Med. Assoc.* 267 (1992):2233.

20. L. Alexander, "Medical Science Under Dictatorship," *New Eng. J. Med.* 242 (1949):44.

21. D. C. Thomasma and G. C. Graber, *Euthanasia: Toward an Ethical Social Policy* (New York: Continuum, 1990), 174–78. For a description of the progressive steps in the involuntary taking of life in Nazi Germany, see J. D. Arras, "The Right to Die on the Slippery Slope," *Social Theory and Practice* 8 (1982):297; Rachels, *End of Life,* 175–78; Burgess, "The Great Slippery-Slope Argument," 169–74.

22. R. J. Lifton, *The Nazi Doctors: Medical Killing and the Psychology of Genocide* (New York: Basic, 1986), 14. Lifton is careful to distinguish euthanasia in the traditional Western sense from the Nazi version, adopted to make the party's activities sound acceptable.

23. M. P. Battin, "Fiction as Forecast," 119.

24. "The Right to Die," *Economist,* September 17, 1994, p. 14.

25. C. S. Campbell, "Aid-in-Dying and the Taking of Human Life," *J. Med. Ethics* 18 (1992):128–34.

26. I am indebted to Edwin C. Cadman, M.D., professor of medicine and chief of Staff, and John McNeff, administrative director for finance, Yale–New Haven Hospital, for discussing the financing of health care with me.

27. D. Orentlicher, "Paying Physicians to Do Less: Financial Incentives to Limit Care," *U. of Richmond Law Rev.* 30 (1996):155–97.

28. E. J. Emanuel and L. L. Emanual, "The Economics of Dying: The Illusion of Cost Savings at the End of Life," *New Eng. J. Med.* 330 (1994):540–44.

29. T. Bodenheimer, "The HMO Backlash: Righteous or Reactionary?" *New Eng. J. Med.* 335 (1996):1601–4.

30. S. A. Schroder, "The Medically Uninsured: Will They Always Be With Us?" *New Eng. J. Med.* 334 (1996):1130–33.

CHAPTER 7   THE LEGAL BASIS FOR ASSISTED DYING

Epigraph: This quotation is engraved on the wall of the Jefferson Memorial in Washington, D.C.

1. Justice Oliver Wendell Holmes commented on outdated laws: "It is revolting to have no better reason for a rule than that it was laid down at the time of Henry IV. It is still more revolting if the grounds upon which it was laid down have vanished long since, and the rule simply persists from blind imitation of the past" ("The Path of the Law," *Harvard Law Review* 1887: 457–69).

2. G. S. Neeley, preface to *The Constitutional Right to Suicide: A Legal and Philosophical Examination* (New York: Peter Lang, 1994).

3. Justice Douglas in *Griswold v. Connecticut,* 381 U.S. 479, 484 (1965).

4. *Palko v. Connecticut,* 302 U.S. 319, 324–26 (1937).

5. Justice Brennan in *Carey v. Population Service International,* 431 U.S. 678, 684–85, quoting *Whalen v. Roe* 429 U.S. 589, 599–600 (1977).

6. *Cruzan v. Director, Missouri Department of Health,* 497 U.S. 261 (1990).

7. The legality of assisted suicide is unclear in Iowa, North Carolina, Utah, Virginia, and Wyoming. Assisted dying is now legal in Oregon.

8. *Compassion in Dying v. State of Washington,* 79 F.3d 790, 824 (9th Cir. 1996).

9. Justice Goldberg in *Griswold v. Connecticut,* 381 U.S. 479, 494 (1965).

10. Justice Brandeis in *Olmstead v. United States,* 277 U.S. 438, 478 (1928).

11. *Roe v. Wade,* 410 U.S. 113 (1973).

12. D. P. Judges, *Hard Choices, Lost Voices: How the Abortion Conflict Has Divided America, Distorted Constitutional Rights, and Damaged the Courts*

(Chicago: Ivan R. Dee, 1993). This book provides a detailed review of the events leading up to and following *Roe v. Wade.*

13. Ibid., 103–9.

14. H. Wolinsky and T. Brune, *The Serpent on the Staff* (New York: G. P. Putnam's Sons, 1994), 179–80.

15. *Webster v. Reproduction Health Services,* 492 U.S. 490 (1989). For details of the case see Judges, *Hard Choices,* chapter 14.

16. *Planned Parenthood of Southeastern Pennsylvania v. Casey,* 505 U.S. 833 (1992). For details see Judges, *Hard Choices,* chapter 19.

17. *Planned Parenthood v. Casey,* 505 U.S. at 833 (1992).

18. *In re Quinlan,* 348A 2d 801 (N.J. Super Ch Div., 1975), rev'd., 70, 355 A 2d 647, 662–63 (N.J. 1976).

19. American Medical Association Council on Scientific Affairs and Council on Ethical and Judicial Affairs, "Persistent Vegetative State and the Decision to Withdraw or Withhold Life Support," *J. Am. Med. Assoc.* 263 (1990):426–30; Multi-Society Task Force on P.V.S., "Medical Aspects of the Persistent Vegetative State," *New Eng. J. Med.* 330 (1994):1499–1508, 1572–78.

20. See *Superintendent of Belchertown State School v. Saikewicz,* 370 N.E. 2d 417, 426–27 (Mass. 1977); *In re Conroy,* H.2d 1209, 1236 (N.J. 1985); *Bouvia v. Superior Court,* 179 Cal. App. 3d 1127 (Ct. App. 1986); *Brophy v. New England Sinai Hospital,* Me. Mass. 417, 497 N.E. 2d 626 (Mass. 1986).

21. *Cruzan v. Director, Missouri Department of Health,* 497 U.S. 261 (1990).

22. *Compassion in Dying v. State of Washington,* 79 F.3d 790 (9th Cir. 1996).

23. Ibid.

24. U.S. Court of Appeals of the Ninth Circuit, *Compassion in Dying v. State of Washington,* 79 F.3d at 813–14, quoting *Planned Parenthood v. Casey,* 505 U.S. at 851.

25. *Cruzan v. Director, Missouri Department of Health,* 497 U.S. at 278.

26. *Compassion in Dying v. State of Washington,* 79 F.3d at 812.

27. *Quill v. Vacco,* 80 F.3d 716 (2d Cir. 1996).

28. Circuit Judge Calabresi, in *Quill v. Vacco,* 80 F.3d 742.

29. Justice Brennan in *Carey v. Population Services International* 431 U.S. 678, 684 (1977), in ruling on the sale of contraceptives to people under sixteen years of age.

30. Justice Blackmun, dissenting, *Bowers v. Hardwick,* 478 U.S. 186, 199 (1986), quoting *Olmstead v. United States,* 277 U.S. 438, 478 (1928) (Brandeis, J., dissenting).

31. M. M. Handelsman, "Federal Policy Regarding End-of-Life Decisions," in *Euthanasia: The Good of the Patient, the Good of Society*, ed. R. I. Misbin (Frederick, Md.: University Publishing Group, 1992), 201–14.

32. *Washington v. Glucksberg*, 117 S.Ct. 2258 (1997), and *Quill v. Vacco*, 80 F.3d 716 (2d Cir. 1996).

33. R. Dworkin, "Assisted Suicide: What the Court Really Said," *New York Review of Books*, September 25, 1997.

34. S. M. Canick, "Constitutional Aspects of Physician Assisted Suicide after *Lee v. Oregon*," *Am. J. Law. and Med.* 23 (1997):69–96.

35. I am indebted to Professor Michael Reisman of Yale Law School for discussing these aspects of the law with me. In this analogy, I use the terms *hard* and *soft law* in ways that are different from how they are used in international law, where they were coined. As Professor Reisman explained to me, *soft law* refers to principles like modus vivendi, which establishes appropriate behavior for each of the parties to it but can be denounced by either party without notice or on very short notice. *Soft law* also refers to guidelines that do not have sanctions for their violation or mechanisms for their enforcement. From a proper legal point of view, my discussion is more in the order of an operational code than of soft law.

36. W. M. Reisman, *Folded Lies: Bribery, Crusades, and Reforms* (New York: Free Press, 1979).

37. W. J. Winslade, "Physician-Assisted Suicide: Evolving Public Policies," in *Physician-Assisted Suicide*, ed. Robb Weir (Bloomington: Indiana University Press, 1997), 233.

CHAPTER 8. FROM PATIENTS TO PHYSICIANS AND POLICY

Epigraph: "Prolonging Life, Permitting Life to End," *Harvard Magazine*, July–August 1995, pp. 46–51. Francis Moore is the Moseley Professor of Surgery at Harvard Medical School and former chief of surgery at the Peter Bent Brigham Hospital, Boston. He is one of the most highly respected educators in American medicine.

1. W. Gaylin et al. "Doctors Must Not Kill," *J. Am. Med. Assoc.* 254 (1988): 2139–40.

2. P. A. Singer, M. Siegler, "Euthanasia: A Critique," *New Eng. J. Med.* 322 (1990):1883.

3. D. Orentlicher, "The Legalization of Physician Assisted Suicide: A Very Modest Revolution," *Boston Col. Law Rev.* 38 (1997):443–75.

4. D. Callahan and M. White, "The Legalization of Physician-Assisted Suicide: Creating a Regulatory Potemkin Village," *U. of Richmond Law Rev.* 30 (1996):24, 63.

5. E. Emanuel, "Whose Right to Die?" *Atlantic Monthly,* March 1997, pp. 73–79.

6. "Mercy for the Dying," editorial, *New York Times,* May 28, 1994.

7. R. F. White, "Physician-Assisted Suicide and the Suicide Machine" in Misbin, *Euthanasia,* 196.

8. S. Jamison, *Final Acts of Love: Families, Friends, and Assisted Dying* (New York: G. P. Putnam's Sons, 1995). This book details many aspects of decision making and communication by dying patients and families and physicians.

9. S. T. Murphy et al., "Ethnicity and Advance Care Directives," *J. of Law, Med., and Ethics* 24 (1996):108–17.

Index